Curiosity Heals
the Human

How to Solve "Unsolvable" Medical Challenges With Better Questions and Advanced Technologies

By David Haase, MD
#1 Bestselling Author

Acknowledgements

I AM INDEBTED TO:

Janet Haase - you above all

Will, Alex & Katie
Vern & Arlene Haase
Jeff Bland
Deborah German
Sidney Baker
Helen Messier
Brian & Stephanie Blackburn
The Entire MaxWell Clinic® Team
Dan Keuning
Dan Sullivan
Howard Urnovitz
Lee Hood
Vik Chandra & John Q. Walker
Mark Percival & Rick Perryman & Greg Kelly
Todd Lepine & Kara Fitzgerald
Mark Hyman & Patrick Hanaway
Kristi Hughes & Dan Lukaczer
David Perlmutter & Terry Whals
Craig Venter & Peter Diamandis
Randy Buitikofer
Ed Rush & Mike Koenigs
Katie Gutierrez & Corey Blake

Dedicated to all of my patients over the years.

You have been my best teachers.

Thank You.

"I would rather have questions that can't be answered than answers that can't be questioned."

— Richard Feynman

About the Cover

Tensegrity structures are the mascots of Systems Medicine.

Systems are hard to visualize, but you can hold a Tensegrity Structure in your hand. These amazing structures of compression and tension were popularized by Buckminster Fuller, below.

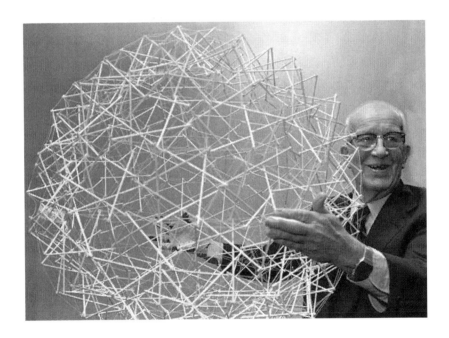

Tensegrity structures have to be held and played with to be appreciated – they are amazingly strong, resilient, complex, beautiful wonders of structure-function. Much like the human body.

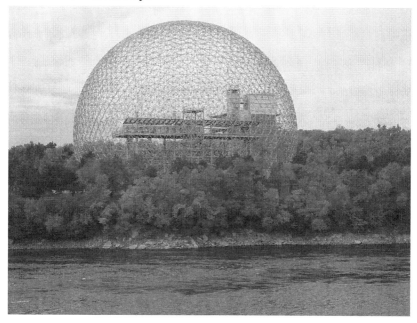

Tensegrity structures are like humans in the following ways:
- It is clear that in both cases the whole is greater than the sum of its parts.
- It is Connection that holds it together – the more connections present, the more stable and resilient the structure.
- They are both Strong, Adaptive, and Resilient.
- They are both not easily understood in 2-D – tensegrity structures are 3D and the number of dimensions or perspectives in which you can describe a human is nearly limitless.

- Each looks different depending upon your angle of perspective.

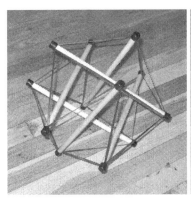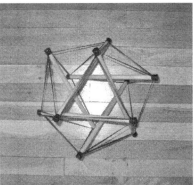

The Tensegrity structure has become my own mascot and it follows me everywhere and reminds me to think SYSTEMS. For more information and musings and a place to get your own pet tensegrity structure, visit us at www.DrHaase.com/tensegrity.

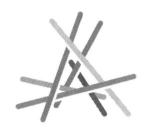

DR.HAASE

Disclaimer

I want you to experience the highest level of health possible – what I call maximum wellness.

I am rather certain the insights in this book can help you to see your health differently and will enable you to ask better questions to improve your outcomes. I wrote it that you may be educated, inspired, and supported towards higher levels of health.

That being said, <u>let me be clear that nothing in this book is meant to substitute for medical advice. I am a physician, but I am not your physician, and nothing in this book is intended to diagnose or treat you in particular for any disease.</u>

I strongly encourage you to develop and deepen a personal doctor-patient relationship with a physician that can walk with you on this journey of creating health. Dive deeply into your markers of health, be aware of and correct early dysfunctions that lead to disease. Share your thoughts and decision making with her or him to obtain the best possible outcomes as you make ever better choices.

Table of Contents

Part 2: Growing a Better Brain

The Center of it All

Ruts & Furrows

The Curious Brain

Part 3: Using Questions to take on Dementia, Data and Cancer:

Curiosity Heals
the Human

Foreword: Curiosity Killed the Cat

"When you stop learning, stop listening, stop looking and asking questions, always new questions, then it is time to die." – Lillian Smith

The greatest threat against your health and happiness is surprisingly your own brain. It rules above all.

In over 20 years of caring for patients in academic centers, mission fields, emergency departments, and clinics, I've found this to be true. One very important reason for this is because one critical ingredient needed for healing can only come from the brain... Curiosity.

I submit that it is curiosity that heals the human, and its lack is a remarkable predictor of needless suffering, disability, loss of independence, and early death.

Curious patients continue to ask: **Why am I not better? How much better could I be? What could be the problem? Who can help me? What can we try next? Is there another test? Is there another treatment? Is there another doctor?**

Doctors range in their levels of curiosity just as patients do. I have learned that not all clinicians appreciate curious patients as much as I do. A curious patient can ruin a tight clinic schedule, and a curious patient can make a doctor who is well learned in his or her field feel threatened and challenged at a level that makes them uncomfortable.

Cat videos. We all love them. Even dog people. Why did curiosity kill the cat? Because cats have wimpy prefrontal lobes. The prefrontal lobe is an area of the brain that controls how we inhibit information. It gives us that space in between stimulus and response.

Cats chase after a laser pointer forever. Cats continue to crawl on the ground when there's Scotch tape on their back and not get used to it. Cats have a seemingly endless interest in putting their heads in tight places, knocking objects off the wall to see what happens, and getting freaked out at almost nothing. Cats are curious to the point that they endanger their own lives.

Dogs, on the other hand, have well-developed prefrontal lobes. A well trained dog can sit at attention while a treat is placed on his nose. He can suppress his desire to chomp at that treat until he is told to do so.

Humans have the most remarkable prefrontal lobes of all mammals. Our prefrontal lobes give us the ability to govern our curiosity so that we are served by it and not destroyed by it. Yet, just as every strength becomes a weakness at the extreme, our brain's desire to make sense of the world often leads to the development of premature conclusions that hinder us from achieving our full potential. The resulting deficiency of curiosity neuters our ability to escape the confines of our past understandings of the world, our health, and ourselves.

This deficiency of curiosity imprisons us in our own brain. Thankfully, it is a prison that can be escaped through the power of questions.

As we will explore more fully in the following chapters, asking more and better questions is fundamental to our pursuit of health. While it may true that curiosity can kill a cat, it is an essential key to healing a human.

Introduction

"Asking the right questions takes as much skill as giving the right answers." – Robert Half

I am so thankful you picked up this book. The act of doing so already demonstrates you are likely the kind of person this book was written for – you desire better answers to the riddle of **What Creates Health?**

You live in a world with more answers than ever before. Instead of creating peace in your mind those answers paradoxically create the need for even better questions.

Questions are powerful, scary things. Questions set our brain to the task of solving and our brain will do whatever it takes to bring resolution to the question at hand. It will work on the task when you think all is quiet, even while you sleep. Questions shape your reality and what you think is possible. Questions cause your mind to focus on one goal over another.

There are questions that shaped my life as a South Dakota farm boy. **Is there a better way?** is one that still rings in my ears. I was born into a family of practical innovators in an environment where all the work of the day was on your own shoulders. There was great value in finding the most true and efficient way to go about any task. The better we followed natural laws and principles in general, the more our crops and livestock flourished. The question, "Is there a better way?" continues to be front and center as I go through my day as a physician-innovator.

In college, I began to experience life outside of the farm but questions remained important to me. For example, while working in a leper colony in Nigeria, I recall again being changed by a question – **What is the purpose of pain?** You see, leprosy is an infection that affects the pain-sensing nerves in the body. The longer the infection rages the more nerve fibers are destroyed, decreasing the patient's ability to feel pain. All it takes is one pebble in a shoe plus a stroll down the road, and a massive painless injury could occur and progress to infection and loss of the foot. The same thing happens when a person reaches out to move what was thought to be a cool kettle – no pain as the flesh is seared. No withdrawal reflex from the pain.

Pain, like every other symptom, is there to inform us of dysfunction. Pain has a built-in intent to help us identify the offending culprit causing the pain so that we can remove that cause. Pain presents a question to the brain that demands an immediate answer in the form of a protective reflex. This question of the purposefulness of pain shaped my clinical mind to embrace symptoms as informational gold in finding the root causes of disease. An opportunity to ask **Why?** and to solve a riddle.

There is a time in life when all of us share a passion for questions. What three year old has not played the 'why' game? "Why do I have to go to bed?' / 'Because you need your sleep.' / 'Why do I need my sleep?' / 'So that your body can grow big and strong.' / 'Why does my body need to grow big and strong?' / 'So that you can play with your friends and have fun.' / 'Why should I play with my friends and have fun?" and on and on and on. Parents usually surrender with, "Just because," or "Someday you'll understand."

As a physician nearing 50, I'm still playing this game. I am a perpetual three-year-old... and I suspect you may be as well. I have one word I just can't quit asking that has frustrated, exasperated, and even infuriated "experts" in the realm of medicine for years. That word is **Why? Why does disease occur? Why can two people with nearly identical lifestyles have such different health outcomes? Why is our healthcare system focused on treating disease rather than creating health? Why does wholesome innovation take so long to be incorporated into clinical practice?** And the list goes on.

Often times the more "expert" an individual, the more disturbed he or she is when a question is posed by a learner – especially if the learner continues to follow-up the initial answer with another round of "Why?" We will discuss the neurology of this phenomenon later.

Incessantly asking **Why?** is the essence of root-cause analysis, and the best route to finding meaningful solutions to our most persistent problems of today.

There is no place where asking better questions is more critical than when it comes to our health and well-being.

Today, that smartphone next to you gives you access to the world's knowledge on health, and any other conceivable subject. But when I was choosing the medical school I would attend, a major determinant used by those who rank medical schools was the size of the library. How many issues of ancient periodicals that were stored in the bowels of the heart of the school determined how much access you had to accumulated knowledge.

I remember having a question, going to the library, feeling like hot stuff because I had access to a database of medical terms stored on a non-networked computer (the Indicus Medicus), writing down my results on an index card, looking up the location of the journal in the building, searching it out in endless rows of bound periodicals, paging to the reference, and ultimately deciding if it was worth the 5 cents a page to photocopy. If it was worthy I would highlight and store it in a growing file cabinet system – because the mark of a great scholar at that time was how quickly you could find just the right article to prove your point.

Now I (and anybody else in the world) can just say, "OK Google," "Hey Siri," or "Alexa..." and ask a complex medical question and get an answer much faster than a half-a-day in the library struggling with Index Medicus.

We are overwhelmed with answers – competing answers – conflicting answers. And no-more-so than in the realm of health and disease with the fickle Doctor Google always willing to diagnose us with some horrible condition or a Facebook "friend" or self-promotional blogger selling us the never-before-known-to-man super-simple magic solution to all our health problems.

With the advent of artificial intelligence, we will have more and better answers than ever before. But always, the quality of our questions will determine the quality of the answers we receive. Ask the wrong question and the answer you receive – while it may be accurate and timely – will be at best useless, and at worst deceptive, encumbering, and dangerous.

Try the following exercise: Think about a diagnosis that has great importance to you – one that either currently or in the past has challenged you or a family member. If you can't think of one, use Alzheimer's dementia, as it is now the <u>leading cause of death in the United Kingdom</u>[1]. Now, mentally place that diagnosis in the area below.

---

[1] https://www.theguardian.com/society/2016/nov/14/dementia-and-alzheimers-leading-cause-of-death-england-and-wales

I (or my loved one) have just been diagnosed with

_____.

The name of a disease when given to a patient as a diagnosis is an *answer*. And an answer is a problem when it implies that it is the final word. All good scientific answers create more questions than they solve. A diagnosis – like depression, dementia, or diabetes – should not simply be an answer. Rather, a diagnosis should be a place to start asking questions and to start asking better questions.

I contend that the phrase, "I have ___ (insert diagnosis here) _____" is not the best way to understand reality as it relates to health and disease. What we call "Diabetes" or "Depression" or "Alzheimer's," we now understand to be the complex and unfortunate end results of multiple genetic-environmental interactions accumulated over time.

Instead of saying, "I have Diabetes" as a statement of end fact, think how useful it could be to say, "I currently have a diagnosis of type 2 diabetes which was likely caused by _____ and _____ and ____ and _____ interacting together over time." Those 4 blanks represent 4 or more opportunities to potentially halt or reverse this process. How does one find what fits in those blanks? Curiosity!

A diagnosis should always mark a new beginning of inquiry, not the end of questioning.

In many medical settings, we have learned to ask only one question after receiving a diagnosis:

What drug can fix _____**?"**

This question, "What drug can fix...?" isn't always conscious. But it is the implied question you are asking IF you seek care from a medical provider that is content to label your complex situation with a diagnostic code (required for billing purposes) and has pharmaceutical treatments as the only tool in the box.

What different kinds of answers would you expect from the following statement and questions?

"My health is not what I desire. What could be the underlying causes of my current state of health, and how can I change my situation?"

The more we understand in science, the more surprising it is how many avenues there are to health and disease. When we ask better questions, and investigate more deeply, we find some remarkable answers for the individual.

One new approach to searching for better answers to our question of underlying causes of disease comes from the world of "omics."

An "Ome" is a suffix that is applied to words to describe all the parts of a system and all the interactions of a system. Data of this richness is both an answer and an engine for better questions

Searching through this complex set of data to find practical solutions for the patient is the domain of Personalized Systems Medicine. Our many systems of genome, microbiome, exposeome, nutriome, connectome, metabolome, ideome, etc. all interact together to create the health situation we have.

Said more succinctly – we are complex beings that can be understood in new and more complete ways every day. We have a remarkable capacity for thriving and we deserve better than dumbed-down, overly-simplified answers to our very real and complex problems of disease and dysfunction.

Better questions will help us find better answers.

As I share with you some of the most powerful questions I have encountered in my path as a leader in Personalized Systems Medicine, I will also share some of the answers and deeper questions I have found to be the most surprising and potent as I have treated patients with dementia, diabetes, cancer, depression, autoimmune disease, anxiety, irritable bowel syndrome, and others.

This book is divided into five parts. The first section lets you into my head – where we will journey together on my rather obsessive quest to figure out "What Creates Health?" The second part will give you new insight into how to better understand and optimize your brain, and what major adversary you will need to conquer to be successful. The third section puts questions into action and reveals some of our ground-breaking work treating neurodegenerative disease in particular. Part four dives deeper into issues of understanding nutritional supplementation and some innovative tools for greater success against cancer. And the final section will give you a roadmap for choosing your care team and propelling your health forward.

In short, in this book I will be answering all the important questions.

I just wrote that to see if you were paying attention. Of course not. I will only be scratching the surface. Because a good question leads to an answer that creates more and even better questions! It could feel like work, but your brain is doing this anyway – it is always asking questions like, "How can I be more comfortable? What is there to eat? Should I continue this relationship? What should I wear?" etc. So let us put part of that time towards asking new intentional questions and getting different answers because Curiosity Heals the Human.

Part 1: Curiosity to Creating Health?

Tina is Dead

"Any knowledge that doesn't lead to new questions quickly dies out: it fails to maintain the temperature required for sustaining life." – Wislawa Szymborska

Tina lay dead in her hospital bed because of lack of curiosity.

Tina was a well-dressed, well-spoken, well-educated, well-to-do woman in her mid 50's. She came to the emergency room complaining of nearly 24 hours of severe headache, violent vomiting, heartburn, anxiety and dizziness to the point she couldn't stand up straight. She had treated herself at home for what she called a severe migraine by taking her usual migraine medications of Imitrex® and naproxen, but these did not seem to help. She had been getting very little sleep and had been living on red wine, coffee and pizza for the last week due to a project deadline. At the emergency room, a head CT scan showed that her brain looked normal and there wasn't any bleeding present in the brain.

Treatment in the emergency room was not sufficient to decrease her pain, so she was admitted to our hospital neurology service for observation and pain control. She was not my assigned patient, but since I was a medical student on this particular service, I observed her care by others. She was given IV Toradol®, which is an anti-inflammatory, and IV Dilaudid®, a very powerful narcotic. She was given Phenergan® to decrease her nausea and vomiting, yet, even as these symptoms improved, her heartburn worsened. But with the Phenergan® and Dilaudid® on board, she quickly fell into a sleep-stupor.

Over the next two days, she awoke to complain of the persistence of her severe headache and severe burning in her chest. She was given Green Goddess, which is a cocktail of an antacid, phenobarbital, atropine, scopolamine and lidocaine that numbs and relaxes the esophagus, so you don't feel pain, and some more Dilaudid® for her headache. Her anxiety and agitation grew so she was treated with additional Valium® (she said it was one of her regular medications) to aid her sleeping.

Forty-eight hours after being admitted she woke very agitated and complaining of more chest pain than headache. She was given more Dilaudid® and Green Goddess and she, once again, fell asleep. The next time she awoke to rigors, which is a severe shaking of the entire body, and fever with severe chest pain.

At this time, a chest x-ray revealed that she had air in the middle of her chest called the mediastinum and she was immediately admitted to the intensive care unit with a diagnosis of Boerhaave syndrome. Boerhaave syndrome is the rupture of the esophagus that usually occurs in an individual with cirrhosis that has a vomiting episode. Delay in diagnosis can be fatal.

As Tina's condition worsened quickly over the next 24 hours. In the intensive care unit, she was placed on IV fluids, IV antibiotics, medications to keep her heart pumping, and as her lungs quickly filled with fluid she was placed on a ventilator. We learned from her family that she was a chronic alcoholic, had been in treatment several times, and had severe cirrhosis. That information was not given to the doctor caring for her in the emergency room and, per the records, it was never asked.

Within 72 hours of entering the hospital, Tina went into irreversible cardiac arrest and died.

Questioning her prior medical record could have revealed that her anxiety was alcohol withdrawal. Questioning her family or her symptoms could have caused us to suspect cirrhosis. Questioning the severity of her chest pain could have triggered listening to her chest, or getting a chest x-ray sooner. Questioning the onset of her chest pain after recent violent vomiting could have increased suspicion for esophageal rupture.

Every doctor that has cared for sick people over a substantial period of time has watched somebody die because the right question has not been asked. Thinking that doctors are God and should know and anticipate everything is not the point of my story.

The point is that with the **right** questions... Tina may be alive today.

The failure of asking the right questions did not start in the hospital. In the outpatient setting, if she had been working with a doctor that had asked her why she drank so much alcohol, what kind of feelings did it help, when did she start excessive drinking, what were her triggers, what had she found successful to decrease her intake in the past... oh so many questions I still want to ask her.

Diagnostic tests and labs are questions too. Although, not available at that time, I wonder what Tina's qEEG Brain Map would have looked like. I would have wanted want to question her brain: Did it have evidence of an old head injury? Did it have evidence of hypervigilance markers consistent with PTSD? Did she bring in visual and auditory information faster than she could process that information leading to a feeling of being chronically overwhelmed? Was her migraine visible on the brain map as a high-beta or high-delta spot indicating an island of electrical inefficiency? If we could have treated her with neurofeedback could we have eliminated her migraines and decreased her anxiety, as well as her perceived need for alcohol as we have done for other patients?

Did she have early childhood trauma? Other life trauma for which she was doing her best to live through?

What if we asked her about her trigger foods and encouraged avoidance? Her diet for the week preceding is what I would recommend eating if you want to put yourself at high risk of not just a headache, but so many more problems. Red wine, tomato sauce, aged cheeses, and sausage are all foods classically high in histamine and often trigger migraines, especially in patients with increased intestinal permeability. Was this food-borne histamine augmented by alcohol's effect of causing increased release of histamine, and had she developed a deficiency of the enzyme needed to break down histamine (Diamine Oxidase) due to diffuse gut injury as a result of undiagnosed celiac disease? Did she know there was a supplement that could replace Diamine Oxidase until her own gut healed enough to make it on its own?

Did she know that cravings can often be stopped by infusions of specific nutrients? Why did she relapse – was it because of an impairment in her mitochondrial function?

Did anybody ask her what made her feel better and what made her feel worse and then put that into an understanding that could have decreased her symptoms? Was she blown off as somebody who wouldn't change?

Was she menopausal and were her hormones contributing to her problems in the myriad of ways only hormone imbalance can screw someone up? Did anybody assess her for other factors that would have lead to cirrhosis like Glutathione deficiency or fatty liver?

And if she had fatty liver, why did she have that? Did she have a profound magnesium or riboflavin deficiency due to a rotten diet and chronic stress? A genetic mitochondrial disorder? An overgrowth of unhelpful bacteria in her gut leading to increased inflammation and cirrhosis? Deficiency of SAMe causing cellular membrane weakness due to poor phosphatidylethanolamine to phosphatidylcholine conversion and poor intra-membrane protein dynamics? Sorry, nerded out there.

I have often thought about Tina through the years and wondered how her life could possibly have been different. I think about how she could be alive, contributing to the world, pursuing her dreams, and enjoying her grandchildren today. She did not have the chance to do any of these things.

The fact is that Tina had many opportunities for her life to be saved by better questions LONG before she entered the hospital. These questions could have been asked by herself, her doctor, her family, her medical treatment team, or her neighbor. Maybe one of them had the right question.

Tina died for lack of the right questions.

Let this not be the case for you and those you love.

Curiosity Heals the Human.

Dr. German's Question

"Who questions much shall learn much, and retain much."
– Francis Bacon

At Vanderbilt University School of Medicine, my alma mater, the first day of medical school starts with the "White Coat Ceremony." We young doctors-in-training are given our first white coat and are invited into the guild of the medical arts. It is a very emotional time, full of anticipation, excitement, and feelings of responsibility.

It was here that one of the most important questions in my life was asked of me by a mentor I have grown to respect more and more over time. Dr. Deborah German, who was then our Dean of Students, launched into the lecture I most clearly remember from those entire four years. She asked us to tell her what it meant to be *The Good Doctor?*

She waited for us to respond. One by one, we blurted out words and short sentences that spoke from our hearts and heads, words like *compassionate, healer, do-no-harm, knowledgeable, honest, caring, hard-working, dependable, teachable, teacher, decisive, calm, wise, generous, certain, resourceful, leader, skilled, respectable, independent*, and the list went on. What an inspiring vision to cocreate with my fellow future doctors!

I did not realize it at the time, but the lecture lit a fire in me to continue to ask that question of myself. What is *The Good Doctor* as it applies to me in the here and now? As I go through my years as a doctor, I add to this list: *cause-focused, patient-centered, collaborative, function-supporting, upstream, systems-inclusive, brain-honoring*. Each year of medical practice changes my perspective on what it means to be *The Good Doctor*, and how vast the opportunities are for healing.

Knowing the first day of medical school that it was up to me to create and then strive for my own definition of *The Good Doctor* gave me the foundation of freedom and responsibility I needed to grow as a physician.

After Vanderbilt, I moved on to train and practice at the Mayo Clinic in Rochester, Minnesota, where I labored and loved my work, even through the grueling, sometimes hundred-plus-hour weeks.

I trained in family medicine, which may seem a bizarre pursuit at an institution like Mayo which is renowned for its sub-specialties. And an even more bizarre choice coming from Vanderbilt where there wasn't even a department of Family Medicine. Generalism was not emphasized at Vanderbilt, and I was encouraged to seek specialty or subspecialty training by my mentors.

But before coming to Mayo, during my medical school specialty rotations, Tina and patients like her happened. I recognized they all died because in some way *the person* and that person's *life context* had been forgotten in the quest to treat the organ that was the domain of the attending specialist.

I had observed patients die or be harmed due to the brain-bias that is part of being a specialist. You already know about Tina, but there were others.

On a cardiology rotation, while being hospitalized for an abnormal heart rhythm, a patient bled out from a stomach ulcer due to taking chronic ibuprofen for his shoulder pain. He had a history of having ulcers and chest symptoms that went away with antacids, which in retrospect were pretty good clues that he had an ulcer.

On a gastroenterology rotation, a person with a severe flare of inflammatory bowel disease died because his leg swelling was not recognized as new, and a blood clot hanging out in his leg veins went to his lungs, causing immediate cardiopulmonary arrest.

And, on an otolaryngology (ENT) rotation, one of the patients died from an insulin overdose, presumably due to the surgeon overseeing his case being overtired and writing the wrong order in the patient's chart. But I suspect it was instead that the surgical outcome and all things related to the head and neck were more prominent in his mind.

Don't take this the wrong way. I am not anti-specialist, or anti-anything that works for that matter. Many people's lives were and are saved by the brilliance and focus of the organ-focused-sub-specialist. Both Mayo and Vanderbilt are extraordinary facilities with highly competent and compassionate physicians, to whom I refer regularly and trust deeply. People who end up in hospitals are often very complex, and very sick, and often challenged in communication skills. Hospital medicine is very hard medicine, and without it many people would not be alive today.

Yet, those patient experiences were deeply painful for me. For me to be true to my definition of *The Good Doctor* I knew I needed to do what I could to not cause harm via the tunnel vision that I perceived accompanied organ-based-specialization.

An alarming recent study in The Journal of Patient Care[2] estimates that between 210,000 and 400,000 patients die per year as a result of preventable adverse events in hospitals. This would make medical errors the third leading cause of death in the US, following heart disease and cancer. Not

---

[2] James, Patient Saf. 2013 Sep;9(3):122-8. doi: 10.1097/PTS.0b013e3182948a69

only that, but serious harm seems to be 10-
to 20-fold more common than harm that
results in death.

Instead, I saw myself preparing to be someone like my family doctor in Scotland, SD, Dr. Manuel D. Ramos, who knew how to do most of what was needed for patient care. He knew patients as whole people in the context of this community of under 1,000 people. For years, growing up, I saw him know and serve generations of patients within the context of their environment which was obviously and inextricably woven into the fabric of their health.

Most important to me, he embraced my curiosity and took delight in my questions. Every time I had a malady of some sort – an appendix ready to burst, a concussion from falling down the stairs, many bouts of strep throat which earned me an eventual tonsillectomy – he took care of me. But more than that he asked me questions, and quizzed me on the workings of the human body. It gave both of us delight when I could recite back his immunology lecture given to me during the hospital rounds on me the previous morning. He even invited me to scrub in and assist him in the operating room when I was but a junior in high school. Nothing inspires curiosity of what creates health like seeing and putting one's hands inside a human body.

With that background and a degree from Vanderbilt Medical School, I began researching and visiting many medical residency programs. I realized that The Mayo Clinic would afford me a great opportunity to learn from world-renowned specialists during my training as a family physician. Plus, I was motivated by the midwestern idea that family doctors (like Dr. Ramos) should strive to be "comprehensivists" – taking ownership of their patients problems to the extent they can, rather than serving mainly as a source for specialty referrals. I liked that idea.

At the Mayo Clinic, everything seemed to be going well – at least on the surface. I enjoyed my patients, and enjoyed the work. I'd become more confident as a doctor and could make good diagnoses and prescribe "by the book" treatments with high efficiency. I thought my results of changing numbers and symptoms were in line with my expectations.

Everything should have been great, right?

Well, increasingly, something felt off.

While in residency, I was one of the founding members of the first *Evidence-Based Medicine* journal club at Mayo. Its purpose was to gather together as medical doctors and better learn how to independently read and interpret primary research rather than rely on dated textbooks or what the older doctors told us do. As we started to rip into medical articles, many of us were shocked and more than a little dismayed by the lack of evidence our prescribed treatments were based upon. Study after study revealed that what we thought was good care was at best ineffective and at worst just plain dangerous.

For example, I remember reviewing the new medication Rezulin® in our club, and the vast majority of the attendees thought it was a breakthrough new treatment for diabetes. Yet, in the study used to approve the drug, many participants had elevated liver enzymes and one had liver failure. I voiced my concern that this drug may do more harm than good. It was not a popular stand I clearly recall.

That was in the spring of 1997. After 2.8 billion dollars in sales, the drug was forcibly removed from the market by the FDA in March of 2001 after at least 65 deaths, dozens of liver failures, and transplants. And it had never shown evidence of life-saving benefit to give some justification for the harm inflicted. Of note, Britain removed the drug from sale in December of 1997. Yes, we have cause to distrust our pharmaceutical industry.

This concern about what we as medical doctors were doing began to seep deeply into me, and I drifted dangerously close to therapeutic nihilism. I strongly considered leaving medicine – but a new baby boy at home and my medical school debt kept me from bolting.

Over time, I increasingly saw the shortcomings of a reductionist approach to medicine – the "naming, blaming, taming" routine. Good treatment was defined by making diagnoses (naming), telling the patient the cause of their problems was the diagnosis (blaming), and then providing medical treatment to suppress a symptom or change a number (taming). All too often at this point, the questioning of *why* this person had dysfunctional health in the first place had ceased or had never been considered.

I became dismayed that one medication I would prescribe would cause a side effect would require another drug to address. Neither of these drugs would fix the underlying cause of the problem, and would instead cause nutritional depletions and metabolic changes leading to more diagnoses and more drugs – the dreaded "prescription cascade." I found that I was not looking for and addressing multiple interrelated causes but rather practicing "one-bug, one-drug" medicine, a philosophy born out of the antibiotic/vaccine revolution and encouraged by our medical coding and billing practices.

I noticed that lifestyle interventions were rarely taught or encouraged in practice and began to see that economics shaped medicine more than I wanted to admit. For example, the more complex the visit, the more a doctor can charge for that visit, and prescribing a medication rather than recommending a lifestyle change increased the "complexity." It naturally followed that since lifestyle recommendations did not count as complexity, and because good counseling takes time in an office visit, spending the time exploring bigger picture solutions was not something that the system economically encouraged.

I increasingly came to understand that our standard-of-care was reductionist medicine which unintentionally carved people up into organs and tissues and symptoms and treated with more-dangerous than needed interventions all too often.

I want to be clear that the physicians with whom I worked at Mayo and Vanderbilt were and are some of the finest people I have ever known. Caring, thoughtful, wickedly smart and masters of their art. I knew I was training with the best of the best in the world; yet, I did not know where to turn for a perspective that took into account the complexity of causation. Everything was in pieces – individual diagnoses – multiple sub-specialists – disjointed therapies that often worked against each other. It was driving me nuts and making me question my life's calling. I could hear the question of Dr. German in the background, "What is *The Good Doctor?*" and I wasn't feeling it was me.

Crazily enough, during my time at the Mayo Clinic, I had what I can only call a conversion experience that would forever change my life and practice. I encountered a brilliant biochemist, Dr. Jeffrey Bland, at a continuing medical education event in Montana, on the topic of "Food as Medicine." I'd signed on mainly for the advertised gourmet food and because it took place in the mountains. But when Dr. Bland took the stage and began to speak, I felt as if I was the only person in the room and he was speaking directly to me. Through his new curiosity-driven perspectives, I began to find some of the missing pieces and knew that I was in for a lifetime adventure with the complex and beautiful puzzle of health.

Dr. Bland eloquently expounded that medicine as it is currently practiced is organized within a linear system. (Once again, *one-bug-one-drug*.) In our excitement to find single-drug cures, we were lured by the siren call of reductionism: the belief that we can study human health like we can study how billiard balls bounce when they collide, or the belief that health problems are simple and can be effectively treated by single-action solutions to suppress symptoms and "manage disease." This linear line of thought is convenient for pharma sales, bean-counters and medical billing, but it does not adequately describe the human experience.

Dr. Bland asked the questions – **"How should our System optimally function? and What can be done to improve that function?"** These questions take us back to focusing on health rather than disease as we seek to understand the process of how we become well.

At the conference, Dr. Bland used the medical literature to demonstrate again and again that the body is more accurately understood as a complex, dynamic, interactive system of networks, and it is the *functioning* of these interdependent networks that determines human health and disease.

As I saw this literature laid out before me, I realized I did not have to throw out all of my years of medical school and look to Chinese medicine or Ayurveda or some other unifying system of medical theory to proceed as a whole-person doctor! My father-in-law was very happy that I was now content to keep my job and his daughter would not be destitute. Ha!

Through the lens of function, I could simply open my mind to the connectedness of all that I knew and look at the same treasure trove of information in the medical library in a new way. I was on cloud nine, breathing fast and wide-eyed with wonder that the shift could be so subtle, yet so powerful. But, oh, the implications of looking at the world of health and disease in a new way were enormous – and would greatly disrupt my medical career from that moment on. SO MANY QUESTIONS!

Schooled by Amos

"It's hard for me to ask questions I haven't thought about."
– Ryne Sandberg

Mayo Clinic had provided me with superb, top-tier training as a budding "comprehensivist," and great preparation to fulfill my dream of being a small-town doctor, like my family doctor, Dr. Ramos. So, stethoscope in hand and my family in the car, I set out for rural Iowa and joined a small practice.

At this point on my journey over 20 yrs ago, I'd already had my road-to-Damascus moment with Dr. Jeff Bland and the budding field of Functional Medicine. I also knew that I could have scientific integrity and be holistic as an MD. I had started to implement diet, supplements, and individualized hormone treatment protocols while still at Mayo, but in truth I still felt I was just dabbling.

Was I on board with the idea of finding the underlying cause and assisting the body to heal? Sure! But I hadn't yet seen its effects large-scale with my own patients. While generally disillusioned with it, traditional-style practice hadn't really let me down enough to take on the professional ridicule and effort that a full change-over would induce. That was about to change.

John was a salt-of-the-earth Iowan, forty-six years old, a churchgoer, a husband, a father, worked in manufacturing, grew up on a farm – a decent, kind guy. He was mildly obese, and over the course of a year, I diagnosed him with high cholesterol, GERD (heartburn), diabetes, high blood pressure, depression, and IBS (irritable bowel syndrome). When he first visited my practice, I gave him the usual: I diagnosed and treated, with a lot of medications (Lipitor® for high cholesterol, Prilosec® for acid reflux, Toprol® for high blood pressure, Metformin® for diabetes, and Prozac® for depression). I was practicing medicine by the book, and I was practicing it well as evidenced by John's cholesterol and blood sugar numbers improving. I gave John a good dose of name-it-blame-it-tame-it conventional care.

But after many visits with no improvement in his IBS or depression and a worsening of his fatigue and pain, John decided to see another doctor. When the other guy's treatment worked, John came back to me and let me know about it. What was surprising is that the new "doctor" was an Amish elder who lived nearby whom John had heard of through a friend. John, however, didn't return to deliver the message of success in a spirit of gloating or spite. "I just wanted to let you know I'm better," he said.

It was a wake-up call, a tipping point. Somebody else had succeeded where I failed. *The Good Doctor* can't be offended by such feedback, but I couldn't help being taken aback. How could this have happened? *I'm the one with all this schooling,* I thought, *the trusted source of information, and this Amos hasn't passed the eighth grade in formal education, hasn't taken organic chemistry, can't drive a car, and has no license to practice medicine! How dare he! I am a Mayo Doctor for heaven's sake!* These were my first thoughts, but it didn't take long for my ego to calm down and for me to acknowledge that in the realm of real results, Amos the Amish elder had taken me to school.

Curiosity protected me that day. Without curiosity I would have found a way to ignore John's story, to be distracted by my next task until the unpleasant thoughts got diluted by business. Without curiosity my ego would have won.

I studied John's case from a new perspective and came to grips that <u>I was likely the cause of many of John's problems via "the prescription cascade."</u>

The cholesterol medication lowered his CoQ10 levels and probably raised his blood sugar and contributed to his muscle aches and fatigue; the proton pump inhibitor Prilosec® (the infamous "purple pill") depleted him of vitamin B12 and magnesium which compounded by the CoQ10 and B12 depleting effects of his diabetic medication, Metformin®, could have triggered his depression, and potentially increased his likelihood for hypertension. Prilosec® also decreased his natural and needed stomach acid, which decreased his ability to assimilate minerals, and set him up for abnormal numbers of unfriendly bacteria growing in his bowel, leading to small-intestinal-bowel-overgrowth (SIBO) and irritable bowel syndrome (IBS).

We now know these factors together likely contributed to his anxiety and depression via gut-brain interactions. Further, his blood pressure medication, Metoprolol®, could have directly worsened his depression, worsened his blood sugar, and contributed to additional weight gain.

The Prozac® used to treat his depression was potentially a trigger for fatigue and the symptoms we had labeled as irritable bowel syndrome.

This list of potential detrimental effects of his medications is just from the known effects of the medications when given alone. When you consider the interactions among all five medications John was on, he had the potential for a _nearly unlimited_ set of undesirable effects in his body. My medical school teachers would rant against the dangers of "polypharmacy" and now I had seen it (and created it) firsthand.

The Amish elder listened and asked John what was at the root of his problems – John knew in his heart and his intuition guided the process. Amos suggested John stop all five medications, change his diet, drink only water, walk every day, take some herbs and nutrients, and go to bed earlier. Now John was better. His blood pressure was lower, and his cholesterol levels were good. His mood was bright, and his bowels no longer hurt.

Questions began to flood my mind and I knew I had to practice differently. Thanks for taking me to school, Amos.

The Reluctant Clinic

"To raise new questions, new possibilities, to regard old
problems from a new angle, requires creative imagination
and marks real advance in science."
– Albert Einstein

The questions I heard on the farm throughout my
childhood rushed back to my heart. *Is there a better
way? Is it wise? Will it work?* It wasn't about theory;
it was about what was going to get my patients tangible
results. Realizing results are what matters, and driven by
the discomfort of being called out (albeit kindly) as
ineffective, I committed to putting into regular practice
what I'd been learning for years about functional
systems-based medicine.

Shortly thereafter, I got the confirmation I needed that
this was the path for me. A perfect starting point: a family
friend opened up at a holiday gathering, complaining of
visits to over twenty doctors at many famous institutions
for a case of eczema that had persisted for fourteen years.
She'd tried all sorts of therapies to no avail.

"Well," I told her, "there's this new approach I've been
exploring – would you be interested in seeing if I could
help by looking at your case through the lens of systems
medicine?" This being my first real foray into practicing it,

I was a bit intimidated to go there with a family friend, because I didn't want to fall on my face. I had some doubts, but she was really suffering and I knew I could not sleep well knowing I did not do what I could for her.

I figured *it couldn't hurt.* My desperate friend didn't require much persuasion to agree to it either. I took a relatively comprehensive history from her and completed a timeline describing her decline into dysfunction, then made conclusions as to what her tipping points for enabling health may be.

I first asked her, **"When were you last really well?"** I have learned this question is gold. Most people don't think about their health as having a trajectory or of their dysfunction as having causes. Next, I asked her to tell me about how her bowels function. This was polite company, so she shot me an uncomfortable look – but hey, I'm a farm boy turned doctor – I don't always have the best instinct for tact. She replied that she had heartburn, bloating, and nausea most all of the time. And you guessed it, she was on a slew of medications for these symptoms.

After putting it all together I made recommendations. Then, twelve days after we began treatment my friend called me. She was crying.

Turns out they were tears of joy!

"David, I can't believe it!" she exclaimed. "All of those years I couldn't hold my husband's hand because my eczema was so bad, all of those nights being driven nearly mad by the itching of my palms, all of the doctors, the creams, the pills – and who would have imagined your crazy diet and supplements have cured me in less than two weeks! And I am so *happy!* Is that a side effect of all of this? Thank you, thank you, thank you!"

She recounted that the diseased skin had peeled off, and normal (but thin) skin was underneath – no itching, no bleeding, no cracking. And her bowel function and mood had both improved and have remained in a state of improvement for nearly 20 years since that day.

THAT is what I went to medical school for. I felt like I was beginning to live up to the definition of *The Good Doctor* that was the best fit for me and it felt good.

With the news of our third child on the way we decided to move to Tennessee so our kids could grow up close to cousins and at least one set of grandparents. That was a decision that was well made.

I tried *very* hard not to set up my own practice, which would come with all the hassles of hiring, firing, insurance, and administration. Running a medical practice is very difficult and as a result the number of private doctors has been on decline.

But, there was nowhere else for me to go where I felt I really fit in. If I would have stayed on staff at Mayo my talents at innovation would have been discouraged. If I sought out an academic medical or research position I would have had to deal with the layers of organizational politics that robbs one of effectiveness and the joy or life. If I had joined a traditional practice I would have had to see 5-6 patients an hour, naming, blaming, taming. I would have had less room for curiosity – less time for getting to sleuth for causes. I had to take on all aspects of running a business so I could *make room for curiosity*. So with Leisa, an experienced RN who deeply believed in me and my mission, I started MaxWell Clinic®, and the hassle has been so worth it.

Early successes boded well for the future of MaxWell Clinic®. These encouraging cases prompted me to keep moving forward and to buck the scoffing of peers and the economic challenges of seeing many fewer patients a day.

Early on one young woman with multiple sclerosis left her wheelchair for the first time in three years, re-entered the workforce, and got off disability. We guided an older gentleman with polymyositis – a rare inflammatory disease that leads to weakness, swelling, tenderness, and tissue damage – into remission for the first time in twenty years, shifting him into a high-energy and a nearly pain-free state of being. We were able to reverse disease processes to help patients get off of many medications and have higher function to boot.

These results, and others like them, were addictive for this physician. I wanted more. This experience of getting to fulfill one's oath in a more tangible way I think explains why once doctors "cross over" to systems-based medicine they rarely go back.

Throughout the years I have had the honor to work with many brilliant and caring individuals at the clinic. It is hard for me to call them employees, as they are all part of this family of healing. We encourage laughter, hugs and smiles in our facilities as the human side of healing is profoundly powerful. The therapeutic encounter is so much more than the time in a private room with the doctor - it encompasses all aspects of patient interaction. I give large credit to this MaxWell team for our successes. Without a doubt each of these remarkable humans has a deep passion for seeing our patients experience Maximum Wellness and each of them are transformative forces in the journey.

I believe the journey is the reward, and it is sheer joy to get to travel with such awesome patients and co-workers.

What is Health?

"The more knowledge you get, the more questions you ask. The smarter you get, the more you realize everything can be possible." – Georges St-Pierre

A powerful question that has guided me from the beginning (and also influenced me to choose MaxWell as the name of my clinic) is: **What is Health?** Before we go any further, write your definition of <u>what health is</u> below.

_____

_____

_____

_____

_____

_____

Stephen Covey taught in his *7 Habits of Highly Effective People* that you begin with the end in mind. It is the visioning of your outcome that enables you to make great decisions and good choices as you move forward towards that outcome.

Health is a term that gets thrown around a lot, and it often loses its meaning through dilution. I prefer to replace it with the term MaxWell. MaxWell is a word that came out of my yoga practice. I recognized that there's a paradoxical nature of health. On one hand, there is the *willful*

determination to become the fullest version of one's self –
to continue to strive to get better, faster, smarter, to do
everything necessary, to be determined, exercise
willpower and do whatever it takes to succeed. This **Max**
component of health is represented by the *inhalation*,
where in yoga we open and expand and reach and stretch
and move with intention and determination.

On the dark side – individuals who become stuck in the
maximization mentality often do not enjoy their lives and
struggle with a low sense of satisfaction about their life
experiences. This is a tragedy and certainly not in keeping
with a greater definition of health.

The second part of being MaxWell is the **Well**
component. It is the part of health represented by the
exhalation in yoga, which is a resting into a soulful
surrender, a complete acceptance of where and when and
how you are at this moment and a delicious satisfaction of
your present state of being. Wellness is a mindful part of
health.

Maximizing **Well**ness includes inhaling determination to
be the fullest version of yourself and exhaling relaxation,
acceptance, and enjoyment of the wellness you currently
have. Maximizing Wellness was shortened to MaxWell
and it is how we named the clinic I started in 2003.

Many people call the clinic and ask to see Dr. MaxWell or
patients will ask me, "If you are Dr. Haase, then who is Dr.

MaxWell?" At this point in time I have fun with most of them and tell them Dr. MaxWell is sitting in the chair next to me. After a brief bit the confusion in their expression turns to recognition and with a smile it dawns on them... we are each our own best Dr. MaxWell.

Each of us have the capacity and the responsibility to maximize our wellness. To both endeavor to do everything possible and to enjoy whatever satisfaction that we have at this moment.

Being MaxWell is the optimal state of body, mind and spirit that best helps you fulfill your purpose, pursue your dreams and enjoy the process. It is the definition of health that we have found to be the most useful and wholesome.

How has this discussion changed your view of what health is? How does that change how you may interact with your own healthcare? How do you feel about being Dr. MaxWell? Do you have more to learn to be the kind of Dr. MaxWell you want for yourself?

Think on these questions. They are powerful, indeed.

Finding Why

"I am just a child who has never grown up. I still keep asking these 'how' and 'why' questions. Occasionally, I find an answer." – Stephen Hawking

What are other important questions? What questions set the foundation for a strong doctor-patient relationship and the precedent of exploring your health potential through questions?

Let's try an exercise together. This will be a bit tricky as I am not able to guide you using nonverbal clues and clarifications, but take your time and it will be deeply worth it.

Let's pretend we are sitting together in one of our exam rooms at MaxWell Clinic®, I or one of the great doctors and practitioners we have at our clinic have reviewed your health history, and we have already gotten to know each other a bit. I am now going to ask you one of my most powerful and important questions…

What is your health for?

Now, that may seem an odd question, but think about it for a moment. **What is your health for?** In the space below, write your answer.

_____

_____

_____

_____

_____

___(your first answer)

Now, I would like you to answer the following question. **Given what you wrote in the last answer (<u>your first answer</u>), what is important about that to you?** Add that in the space below.

_____

_____

_____

_____

_____

_(your second answer)

Please do not go on unless you have answered the first and second questions, or you're really going to miss the beautiful part of this exercise.

Now, given what you wrote in the <u>second answer</u>, what is important about that to you? Describe it in the space below.

_____

_____

_____

_____

___ (third answer)

Now, we're going to do this one more time. One more question... **Ultimately, when you deeply consider your third answer, what is ultimately most important about that for you?** What is ultimately most important about your health? What do you want your health for? Write it below.

_____
_____
_____
_____
_____

___(ta dah!)

This exercise is an amazing opportunity for self-reflection. "What is your health for?" triggers in our minds a series of thoughts. Like first of all, thinking it's a dumb question because we haven't been asked it before. "I've never been asked that before, and if I haven't been asked a question before, then it must go into the category of stupid things." Ha! But after the initial pushback we start to think, "Okay, well, what do I want from my life?" because we immediately know upon reflection that our health is necessary for us to discover, enable, and enjoy every aspect of what we're on this planet to do.

Now, let me share some answers I have heard over the years… "I want my health… so I can have more energy," or "so that I can remember how to balance my checkbook," or "so I can remember the places, people, and the important events of my life." Maybe what is important about your health is to feel good and to look good. Maybe this first answer is that my health is for service to others.

All of these are wonderful answers and are powerful in their own right, but then we go to the next level, and I ask you, "Well, what is important about that?" Here, we start to uncover the things that we value. If your first answer was, "I want to have more energy," what's important about having more energy could be that, "I can get up in the morning to make breakfast for my children." Or, "That I can complete a full day's work and contribute to the family." You see, we're getting a layer deeper in what is important to you.

Next, let's ask that question again. Well, what's really important about that for you? Here, we start to get to layers of identity. Usually it's a surface identity. A patient will say, "I want my energy so I can enjoy my grandchildren instead of being exhausted by them." And then I ask, "What's important about that?" and the individual will say, "Well, that's what brings me joy, is to see my grandchildren, and I want to have a positive impact in their lives, and I want them to know their grandmother."

If you say, "I want to be productive in the world and contribute to my family," I ask, "What's important about that?" You could say, "Well, I want my family to be comfortable, and for us to be able to do things together and have experiences that are important to us."

If the individual answers, "I want to wake up and make breakfast for my children," but what's important about that is, "I want to make sure they're nourished and have the best start to their day possible, so that their brains can grow and so they know that they are loved because I have fed them well."

Those things just give me chills writing them. And tears. Yeah, I am deeply moved by the human experience every day. It is such an honor to witness.

But when we go to that final layer, I ask, **"Ultimately, what is most important about your health? What is your health for?"** The answers that come almost always, if adequate reflection is given, go to a place of deep identity. The patient who wants to cook breakfast for a child in order to be a positive influence in their life and nurture them and bequeath love, will say, "It's ultimately important because I'm a parent, and good parents love their children and nurture them, and give them a safe home." This individual is making a statement of identity. "This is why I am here, and I must have my health, so that I can fulfill my created purpose."

To the patient who says, "I need energy so I can be productive in the workforce, so my family could have vacations, and we can have experiences." When asked, "What is *ultimately* most important about this?," this patient may tear up and say, "This is what being a good parent means to me. I want to be a provider. I want my children to have experiences so that they can grow to be wise and loving people and contribute to society and not be narrow-minded because they have never seen nor known anything different from the town we live in."

Then I ask the elderly woman, "What is *ultimately* most important about you having your memory, so that you can enjoy your grandchildren, so that you can influence them and raise them?" It will come out that, "All I am left to do is to pass on love and care and wisdom, and I want to do that most for my grandchildren. This is my time to give back and to make generations become better because of my love and caring. It is who I am."

Those statements bring me to another round of tears as I hear them even in my mind. If you have done this exercise, I imagine you have had some kind of a similar effect. If you rushed through the exercise, please go back and reconsider your answers – it can be life changing.

If you know what your health is for, you have an inexhaustible well of meaning from which to draw energy and inspiration to make any change that is in your capacity to achieve. Will power becomes a thing of the past, because instead of powered by will, you are powered by identity, by the very fabric of your being, by the meaning your life holds. When you are in contact with that level of meaning, everything is possible.

When I work with patients one-on-one, the work we do to set the foundation for why we want health are some of the most profound experiences I have had in my life. I am deeply honored to walk down this path with patients. This is part of the renewed doctor-patient relationship of the next century.

Where the Health Am I?

"Do you ask enough questions? Or do you settle for what you know?" – Byrappa

"The more knowledge you get, the more questions you ask. The smarter you get, the more you realize everything can be possible." – Georges St-Pierre

Medical school and residency taught me to ask the questions, **"What disease does this person have?"** and, **"What is the appropriate treatment?"** Those are good questions to ask, and if your doctor is not asking them, you should probably find another doctor.

However, those are not sufficient questions to achieve MaxWell. If we want a better answer from our brain, we need to ask it a better question, and the better question here is, **"What creates health (or MaxWell)?"** The first time that I thought of that question it was like a conversion experience for me.

I recognized I had been asking insufficiently deep and meaningful questions to assist my patients at the level I wanted to assist them. "What creates MaxWell?" or, "What creates health?" are questions that open our mind to an entirely new set of possibilities. Your turn... what do you think creates Health?

_____

_____

_____

_____

_____

_____

The short answer to, "What Creates Health?" is THE BODY.

We are everyday miracles of complex self-adaptive potential walking around living life while being injured from the inside out and the outside in. Our body must constantly heal the damage as we pour acid into our stomachs during digestion, as we burn fuel inside our cells, as we injure the inside of our bowel as we extract nutrients, as we scrape our skin against the outside world, and insult our lungs with smog and allergens and the reactive and toxic molecule called oxygen. We must heal every moment of every day in every cell.

The intelligence which made the body is what heals the body – we are programed to survive, and even thrive IF SUPPORTED WELL.

It is our body that creates health, that enables function. Understanding that our state of optimal function can be described as MaxWell, we recognize that anything less than fully functional is dysfunction.

We recognize dysfunction in our well-being by symptoms such as not feeling our best, decreased memory, energy, mood, stamina or increased pain and fatigue. We also can know that dysfunction exists by laboratory testing. This is very helpful because often silent biochemical dysfunction precedes any type of symptom. It is imperative in a proactive medicine environment to regularly check your body's biochemistry from multiple angles to find early dysfunction and nip it in the bud with the safest potential intervention possible.

Again, anything less than MaxWell is dysfunction. Once dysfunction has been allowed to proceed unchecked, it progresses to a severity that it deserves its own name, and now it gets called a disease. If it is a disease that is accepted by the current authorities that make the International Classification of Disease code set, it may even get its own ICD-10 code.

If this severe dysfunction called disease is allowed to persist, then we start getting disintegration, literally things falling apart little by little, cells starting to degenerate, tissues degenerating, hopes, dreams, memories. This a process of slow death.

Disintegration leads to eventual disability. Disability is a very challenging state of decreased freedom, increased dependency upon others and increased effort to attain and enjoy the maximum capacity of life possible.

When disability and disintegration continue to proceed, we have death.

Your state of health is best understood as a point on a continuum from MaxWell at one end, to death at the other. Once we recognize that all aspects of our health rest on a continuum of function, we no longer view our health simply as either having a disease or not having a disease. Looking at health through the eyes of function gives us power. It restores our capacity to regenerate. It causes us to ask better questions.

I am always shocked when I share this explanation, because almost every patient looks at me and says, "Oh, yeah, that makes sense." It seems so ridiculous that it has never been taught in a medical school. Nor, to my knowledge, have I heard any of my more conventional colleagues speak of it.

Even so, the medical world is moving quickly away from an isolated paradigm of diagnosing and treating disease and towards a paradigm of creating health via Personalized Systems Medicine.

How Do We Create Health?

"Questions are infinitely superior to answers."
– Dan Sullivan

We now likely agree that health exists on a continuum and we're interested in improving our trajectory towards Maximum Wellness and away from degeneration, disability, and death. And together we are clear that it is the body that heals.

It is the job of the optimal health care system to support the body's ability to heal. To enable our system to optimize, there is one principle and a six step cycle I have found necessary to engage.

The principle is this... to create health:

Do What is Wise and Works.

This guiding pragmatism of the MaxWell Way certainly comes from my upbringing on a South Dakota farm. For that I am very thankful because fewer and fewer people in our modern age get to have the intimate relationship that I did with the earth, work, and community. I knew that it if it was my job getting it done right the first time would save me time and effort in the long run. This has informed this guiding principle.

Do What is Wise and Works can be broken down into four major ideas: *Act Now and Act Big, Intervene Upstream, Choose Least Harm* and *Dedication to Results*.

Do: Act Now and Act Big

To attain new outcomes one needs new actions. "Do" reminds us that without action, and enough action, nothing will change. The time to act is NOW, and the extent of action is as BIG as is useful. The older I get, the more I realize that awareness of our own mortality is a strong incentive to do what it takes and to do it now.

What: Intervene Upstream

Symptoms, Diseases, Degeneration, Disability and Death are all downstream problems with complex upstream causes. Seek to find the "cause of the cause of the cause" and address that. It may be necessary to also do some downstream symptom suppression if the problem is severe, but never do this instead of treating the upstream causes, only in addition to treating the upstream causes.

Wise: Choose Least Harm

There is a guiding principle that has been neglected that we must re-embrace and that is "least toxic interventions first." It is important for us to engage therapies that are going to be effective, but all too often we have forgotten that many interventions carry with them known risks.

The interesting thing about starting a particular therapy is that at the beginning of the therapy you never know exactly what the potential benefit will be. Maybe there will be no benefit, and maybe doing nothing will work just as well. Everything is a probability of improvement.

However, doing something almost always adds to the known probability of risk. Sometimes the risk is certainly worth the potential benefit, such as the surgery necessary to remove an inflamed appendix. Other times it may be less obvious, such as taking a chemotherapeutic agent to treat an autoimmune condition.

I believe strongly that <u>we need to exhaust our least toxic interventions first</u> before we progress to more potentially toxic, costly, or damaging interventions.

This is the "do least harm" principle and if we abide by it, we give food, lifestyle, nutritional supplements, and counseling far more attention as we approach the treatment of chronic non-communicable disease. Being curious about our options and choosing the least harm is a great principle for healthcare and life in general.

Works: Dedication to Results

In my clinic I am fond of saying, "Results are the only things that matter." One of my Investigative Medicine Deep Dive patients even made this into a plaque and placed it on his desk!

How we get there is not as important. If a patient has deeply improved it does not matter to me if it was an herb, nutrient, procedure, diet, IV, drug, exercise, intervention, injection, meditation, stem cell therapy, plasma exchange, insight, belief, or hug that got them there. All I care about is achieving the desired result.

Now for the 6 step cycle. This method works across many types of systems, from economic, to ecological, to computer systems. Like "Do what is Wise and Works," these are principles which help us navigate the complexity and non-reducibility of systems. The process is rather universal – and it's application knows no end of variation or depth.

The 6 steps of the cycle are:
1. Imagine the desired state
2. Examine the present reality
3. Replenish regenerative supports
4. Remove degenerative forces
5. Retrain dysfunctional patterns
6. Reboot set-points and return to Imagine and Examine

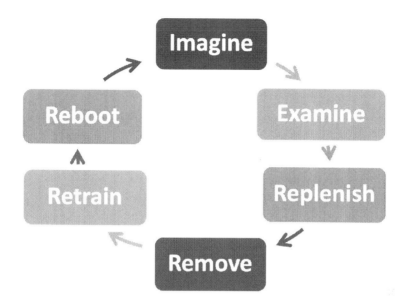

Step 1: Imagine the Desired State

All creation begins in the mind. It is only by thirsting for something more, for something better, that we will put in the effort, energy, time, and money necessary to overcome the inertia of our present circumstances.

Two of my most memorable replies from patients when I asked them what they wanted to accomplish by working together were: "I want to die on my 100th birthday at the hands of a jealous husband!" Oh, that gave me a good laugh – and it communicated that not only longevity was important to this person, but the quality of that life.

The second reply that stood out to me was from a remarkable innovator in this world. Every person reading this book has been touched by this Silicon Valley business and product visionary. This master creator of what-is-next said, "I want to live forever." I had a choice to internally scoff at this reply, but because of the world-changing results this person had already demonstrated in his life, I chose to pause.

In this pause I asked a different question, **"What must be true for my patient to live forever?"** This question changed my life and the entirety of my medical practice. In a large way this question has pushed me to find new solutions for aging, frailty, and neurodegeneration as I will discuss in future chapters.

You can be assured that these bold answers will enable the life these patients desire far more than wimpy answers would. As an expert in longevity medicine I can say that without a big goal, big outcomes are unlikely.

Believe you can be better. Do not settle for the dysfunction that has become part of your current definition of self. Be vibrant, happy, productive, comfortable, and at peace. Do not sell the body-brain short on what it can accomplish. Imagine MaxWell for yourself.

Journaling on the question, **"How will I increasingly feel as I approach my MaxWell?"** will give you a vision of what could be. Jot some ideas here -

_____

_____

_____

Do not underestimate yourself. Over the last 20 years I have seen healing occur that is both dramatic and pervasive. The capacity of the human to regenerate and optimize is incredible – there is no reason the next great transformation will not be you.

Step 2: Examine the Present Reality

The 4th step in a 12 Step program to addiction recovery is to, "Make a fearless and searching moral inventory on ourselves." Alcoholics Anonymous is so successful in part because of this dedication to deep examination of the self.

Likewise, to create health we need to agree to and fully engage in a deep examination of as many aspects of our human system as is possible or practical.

The question that brings wisdom here is, **"What information can I obtain about my body, brain, and behavior that will show me the most potent opportunities for Maximizing Wellness?"**

The extent of this investigation is practically limited by how much money, time, effort, or energy one has available and is willing to dedicate to the journey. These resources are somewhat interchangeable, and more investment of time in learning can shortcut how much energy or effort one must invest. Likewise, more investment into advanced laboratory technologies or expert interpretation can decrease the potential time, energy and effort one would otherwise need to invest to figure out the best plan of action on your own. Sometimes we have an opportunity to choose the type of resources we will invest to create health, but it has been my observation that nobody gets by without investing something of value to receive something of value.

When we reflect upon advanced laboratory testing, we come to realize that Medical Treatment insurance is not built to pay for many of these investigations. This often creates the necessity of a gut-check over what is important, and an honest assessment of how one's resources are invested. It is most important to start where you are with what you have – do not let the best be the enemy of the good. No matter your budget, you can start examining by better listening to your body and asking better questions of your life experience. Questions are free, yet highly valuable for all concerned.

> For those individuals with high resource availability and a dedication to diving deep to address their health concerns and goals, a part of my practice is a Deep-Dive Investigative Medicine program which is detailed later in the book. We start this process with an extensive examination of the reality of the patient's current health state and goals. It includes evaluations of genetics,

metabolomics, hormones, immune function, infectious load, mitochondrial function, nutrient sufficiency, toxin exposure, transport, blood glucose regulation, fatty acid balance, gut microbiome, neurocognitive function, organ reserve and structural measurements, brain MRI with volumetrics, quantitative EEG and other specialized and research-grade testing as appropriate to the patient. We pair this with longitudinal symptom assessments, medical and health history timeline creation, and tracking for lifestyle patterns via wearable devices. A deeper examination creates the potential for a deeper understanding

If we want real results we need to start with as accurate and complete description of your health state at the present time as is possible. Understanding yourself is of tremendous value, especially when this data is integrated into a clinical wisdom engine designed to decipher greater and greater clarity from your health story over the course of time.

Imagination and examination need each other. Imagination enables our mirror neurons to practice our envisioned reality and start the process of change before we move a muscle. Harnessing the power of mirror neurons is why athletes and musicians visualize flawless performances – because it trains their brain to be flawless. Examination keeps us grounded in what is and gives us feedback on real results. With only imagination we suffer delusion; with only examination we suffer stagnation. It is necessary to have both.

Step 3: Replenish Regenerative Supports

We enable the creation of health by replenishing our regenerative supports. I just love the word replenish – it signifies having everything needed, but not being burdened with excess.

We access this knowledge through a question, **"What essential ingredients are inadequate in my life that are needed for me to optimally create health and how do I replenish those?"**

Our body has many nonrenewable resources that are consumed on a daily basis and for the optimal preservation and creation of health. These resources need to be replenished.

At the top of the biological list is **oxygen.** We usually forget about this as our most important nutrient. In my experience, even small degrees of sleep apnea tremendously impact the well-being of the human organism. Slightly less oxygen over a long period of time causes your cellular engines to burn inefficiently. You have all experienced driving behind the car whose carburetor is being subjected to proportionately more fuel than oxygen. The end result is a huge amount of black smoke out the exhaust pipe and a poor fuel to power conversion. That is what happens in our cells if we are insufficiently supplied with oxygen.

Our mitochondria are our internal combustion engines. They take our food, combine it with oxygen, and burn it to make cellular energy called ATP. Carbon dioxide and the cellular soot and smoke comprised of incompletely burned oxygen and fuel is also produced. When this soot and smoke builds up in the system, the cell itself becomes poisoned like a city filled with smog. We call this damage oxidative stress.

The next category of support that is obvious is nutrition. Nutrition has many facets which this brief discussion will not comprehensively cover. In brief, nutrition is comprised of getting enough protein, fat, carbohydrates, minerals, vitamins, and phytonutrients.

I have taught a masters level education course for physicians in human nutrition and to say that there is a lot of detail in this topic is a massive understatement. How we nutrify our body has a massive impact upon the health that we are able to create. Missing just one part on an assembly line holds up the entire factory from fulfilling its purpose. Likewise in the body, a deficiency of one critical nutrient has the effect of gumming up the entire system.

But it's not that simple. Nobody is deficient in just one nutritive material, but rather a complex symphony of nutritional balance is at play in every person.

Let's take fat for instance. Fat has been vilified unjustly by the press as a result of misguided information provided by some healthcare researchers. To speak about fat as a single substance is like speaking about a "vehicle" as a single machine. It is clear a vehicle can be a canoe, a bicycle, a semi, a yacht, a fighter plane, or a Tesla. Fats too have variation to that extent, and details matter greatly.

One of the most important distinctions is the amount of omega-3 fatty acids in the body. This is easily measured by a finger prick at home test. The results have been validated in very large studies and it is clear that levels above 8% of your red blood cells containing omega-3 fatty acids is associated with lower cardiovascular risk rates, lower incidence of dementia and lower all-cause mortality.

I discussed these results with William Harris, PhD, who is a principal researcher involved in a multitude of studies involving omega-3 fatty acids. I asked him, "What is the optimal level of omega-3 fatty acids?" He shared with me that the studies completed were epidemiologic studies. Meaning, they looked at the average amount of omega-3 fatty acids in red blood cells over a large population and then determined the rate of heart disease in those population groups based upon how much omega-3 fatty acids they had in their red blood cells. The challenge was that there were very few people who were in the category of greater than 10% omega-3 fatty acids.

Therefore, it was impossible to make an assessment of whether 10% was better than 8% because so few people were in that category. There has not to my knowledge been a human study has shown a level where too much omega-3 fatty acids in the blood stream becomes detrimental. It is possible, I am sure, because I strongly believe too much of anything can be toxic – but we are nowhere close to getting there with omega 3 fatty acids.

I have recently begun using a very high absorbability Monoglyceride omega-3 fish oil that has enabled my patients to get their omega-3 fatty acid levels up into the 8-12 percent level on a consistent basis. This is Xymogen's Monopure fish oil. I have been astounded at the improvements I have seen with regard to mood, inflammation, and blood lipid panel changes. After over 20 years of using nutrients to improve health and well-being, I am impressed anew by the power of adequately dosed omega-3 fatty acids.

Omega-3 fatty acids are anti-inflammatory, associated with lower cardiovascular risk, and even more remarkably are associated with lower rates of dementia and a seeming improvement in the neurologic function on a large scale. But this only occurs with sufficient blood levels. Some recent popular-press articles have grabbed attention by using headlines suggesting that fish-oil supplements do "nothing". But because the writers only extrapolated off of studies which did not treat towards a goal of optimal omega index, it is not surprising little effect was found. I think these reports are deceptive because we would never claim that ibuprofen did not work for pain if the dose studied was 10 mg (standard low dose is usually 200 mg). As clinician-scientists we know that dosing matters when we are making conclusion about effect. Therefore to make a conclusion as preposterous as the ineffectiveness of fish oil when optimal dosing was not accounted for is to make one wonder what competing interests were involved in such a publication.

Consider asking your doctor about getting an Omega-3 Index, Omega 6:3 ratio, trans-fat and palmitic acid level completed. If you do not have a trusted health professional to work with please visit me at www.DrHaase.com/omega where I plan to detail resources and updates regarding omega-3 fatty acids.

The next major category of nutrients are proteins. Proteins are made of amino acids and amino acids are the building blocks for neurotransmitters, hormones, and all the other structural proteins in your body. If you have a deficiency in one of the essential amino acids, your body has no way to replace this on its own.

So many elderly individuals are protein malnourished and as a result, slowly lose more and more muscle mass. This obvious fact has been seized upon by the food industry with the production of cans of liquid calories with names that speak to reassurance. These literally sickening shakes that are promoted to our elder population are filled with low quality proteins, high amounts of sugar, inflammatory fats, and poorly-absorbable nutrients. Their mere existence just makes me mad. I really believe these cans of swill are doing more harm than good in many cases by convincing folks they are doing a good thing and foregoing real food or at least a high-quality meal replacement shake.

Carbohydrates are sugar molecules that are either single (simple sugars) or arranged in chains (starch or fiber). Carbohydrates are a very important part of a healthy diet and are best consumed as leafy green plant matter and vegetables and whole fruits. When one eats whole foods, many of the other compounds that we're going to talk about next are present at higher levels.

The quality of the food we eat is possibly more important than the type or quantity of food we eat. Seek to eat whole or minimally processed, fresh, local, organic, sustainably raised food whenever possible. It is not just our health we need to be concerned about, but also the health of our planet itself. Conventional farming practices using herbicides and pesticides deplete the soil of microorganisms that add health vigor and nutrient complexity to the soil so the plant can be wholesomely healthy. Organically produced foods increase the number of acres that are not injured by pesticides and herbicides.

One of the questions of curiosity that I find remarkably revealing is, **"What has what I am eating ate?"** This question is applicable if you are eating plants, land animals or fish. Plants from organic land, animals from small farms fed high quality food, fish from clean waters are measurably superior to food that "ate" a sub-standard diet. This translates into my axiom, "You are what you eat has eaten."

Vitamins are "vital amines" which means substances with a nitrogen component that are essential for life. In the biological world, we think of them as cofactors for enzyme function. There are a great variety of vitamin cofactors that are necessary for the metabolism of the body to operate. They are a consumable resource always needing to be replenished.

Minerals have an intimate relationship with enzymes. An enzyme is a complex protein that usually has a mineral in the active site of that molecule. An enzyme enables life to happen by causing chemical reactions to proceed forward in an orderly fashion using the lowest energy possible. When you are mineral deficient, these enzymes do not function at their peak performance; likewise, when you have an abundance of toxic metals in your body, they will usurp these positions in the enzymes and diminish function of the body as a whole.

This is one of the challenges of diagnosing nutritional deficiencies and chemical toxicities; the symptoms and laboratory findings of dysfunction that are produced are subtle and diffuse in the body. If having a zinc deficiency caused your left ring finger to turn green, then it would be an easy diagnosis to make and people would be aware of the problem and the effectiveness of the solution could easily be monitored by the color of your ring finger. But unfortunately, it is not like that.

Nutritional insufficiencies and toxicities cause impaired molecular function, which impairs groups of molecules (called assemblies), which impairs organelles inside the cell, which impairs cellular function, which impairs tissue function, which impairs organ function which finally impairs the function of the organism. So damage at the lower levels is hard to notice, but deeply damaging. Nutritional deficiency is a process of erosion that affects multiple systems slowly. The only treatment is regular repletion of these vital nutrients.

The final category is our phytonutrients. I cannot say enough about the magic of plants. Our bodies function best when we consume a large diversity of plant matter that is in as rough and natural form as is edible. Plants contain fiber, which is a major food source for the healthy population of bacteria that should reside in our gut.

Plants contain many molecules that send messages to our DNA turning on and off genetic patterns in a way that creates remarkable signals for health. These phyto-compounds turn on our antioxidant systems, our mitochondrial repair, our anti-inflammatory responses and our structural repair systems. Brightly colored fruits and vegetables should be the mainstay of our diet regardless of what other tweaking of food components is best for the optimal diet.

I choose to emphasize this with my patients because if you are consuming 7+ cups of a rainbow of colored vegetables and 2+ cups of brightly colored fruits (mostly berries) a day, it's going to be more difficult to eat unwholesomely in the other areas of your life.

Adequate hydration with pure water is another support that we must constantly replenish. Our bodies are water-based organisms and much of our biochemistry exists in an aqueous phase. Even slight amounts of dehydration will cause our enzymes and body systems to dysfunction on a global level. Clean water, preferably that runs through a good filter coming from your tap, is a preferred source. Store this water in glass, stainless steel, or ceramic containers. Try to resist creating more plastic in the world to carry around your water source. I think that the net damage of the plasticizers and contaminants in the plastic may be far more harmful than the chlorinators in our city water sources.

However, I would prefer that you be exposed to neither the plasticizers nor the chlorine and instead use a high quality water filter on your municipal water supply to enable your best health.

Another support that is non-negotiable is activity. Exercise turns on our genetics in a way that produces health and longevity. Just do it – something that brings you joy or pleasure simultaneously would be best. Like all good things, this can be overdosed as well.

Additional supports that the body needs to thrive include full spectrum light. Certain wave forms of light, especially in the morning and evening, in the red light spectrum turn on our body's clock and enable a more restful sleeping pattern. Ultraviolet light causes our skin to make vitamin D. And light intensity itself has an effect on mood. It is profound to consider how many other ways light may affect us that we have not figured out yet. So time spent outside in nature certainly feels good, and is good for us.

Another input or support that we need is sound. It is interesting to note how natural sound such as rain falling on a rooftop is so very different from an unnatural random sound like static. When our ears cannot bring in a particular frequency of sound, this will often be the cause of ringing in the ears, because the body is desiring to have that input into its system.

One of the earliest forms of hearing loss is the inability to understand words in certain frequencies. If this is occurring for you or somebody you love, consider the use of hearing aids quickly because over time if you are not exposed to these sounds your brain will forget what words sound like in those frequencies. Then, years later, when you finally succumb to hearing aids, it does not matter if you turn up the volume of that frequency, the brain has forgotten how to process it effectively and the benefits of the hearing aid end up to be much less than anticipated.

Ultimately, the body craves neurologic input of all types: light, sound, touch, taste, sensation, and what we call proprioception, the awareness of ourselves in space.

We also need each other – the support of community is essential. We exist as members of a community. We need others, not only for our daily sustenance and survival, but we need relationship to align our minds and give us a sense of safety and security. The quality of our relationships is highly predictive of the quality of our health.

We also need quiet. Meditation and mindfulness training are powerful tools to calm the sympathetic nervous system in a way that produces balance and quiets the mind. I have been very impressed with an at-home headset that I have utilized to improve my meditation. It is the Muse headband and it speeds up the process to learn meditation.

Another important support we each need is meaning and purpose in our life. We need a narrative that gives our days and minutes purpose. I've been astounded at how many people feel that their meaning increases by recognizing that the daily engagement of life and becoming the fullest version of themselves is a worthy endeavor. We are each members of an immense community, and have incredibly important roles to play in our families, our workplaces, our nation, and our world. Being the fullest version of yourself is certainly replete with meaning.

Step 4: Remove Degenerative Forces

Next is the removal of degenerative forces. The operative question of curiosity here is, **"What is present in my life and body that is impairing my body's capacity to heal and how do I remove it?"** Degeneration is comprised of all the things that wear us down, break us apart, or injure us. Degeneration and stress can come in many different forms.

There are biochemical stressors such as toxic metals, mold toxins, chemical toxins, radioactive substances, pharmaceuticals, pesticides, herbicides, excess calories, free oxygen radicals, and a multitude of toxic metabolites your body makes on a daily basis. All of these need to be compensated for and detoxified.

In our land and oceans, we unfortunately find these residuals of humanity. I used to be a strong advocate of eating cold water fish as a very important health behavior.

Now I am concerned that eating large sea fish other than Alaskan wild-caught salmon may be too toxic to have a net benefit over harm (I now advocate much more strongly for certified-purity fish oil capsules). That may be a controversial statement at this moment, but unfortunately I will be proven right over time.

Psychological stress is often what we mean when we use the word stress. This includes the feeling of being tense or overwhelmed, and the challenges that we may feel from changes taking place in our world – be that a new job, a new relationship, or a change in our understanding of who we are.

Electromagnetic stressors are not often considered, but are always present. The waveforms of light and sound as they invisibly occur around us influence our health. This is easy to experience. All one needs to do is to walk outside of the fluorescent cave we humans call an office into the sunshine and somehow your body knows that outside is just more wholesome than inside. We have much to learn in this domain and the fact that we cannot see energy and electromagnetic patterns should not decrease our curiosity about their effect upon our health.

Another type of stress is immunologic. Our immune system is our department of defense. It is designed to protect and restore us. It fights against microbes, toxins, viruses, bacteria, fungi, molds, and keeps us alive. Unfortunately, our immune system can turn on us and create autoimmune disease. When this occurs, our body begins to fight against itself and creates the damaging force of inflammation.

We often encounter structural stressors such as injuries to tissue or a twisted knee, a clogged sinus passage, or the residual effects of poor alignment of the spine as one exercises heavily. Sitting has been called the new smoking because it has such detrimental effects on our health. We wouldn't typically think of sitting as a stressor but it certainly qualifies.

Let's go a little deeper into an exposure that is usually a daily occurrence. Could your food be a degenerative force?

I will always remember the first time I heard Dr. Sidney Baker, the poet laureate of functional medicine, state his law of the tacks. It goes something like this, "If you're sitting on a tack, it takes a lot of aspirin to feel better." This signifies the truism that if you have something in your system that's irritating you, is causing dysfunction, pain, and lack of joy, it is wise to remove that thing if you desire health.

Just taking a suppressing substance (drug), or distracting yourself, or denying that it is a problem is not the wisest course of action. The best course of action is to find the offending cause and remove it.

Dr. Baker had a corollary to the law of the tacks. "If you're sitting on two tacks, removing one doesn't make you 50% better."

This is obvious upon reflection. If you have two irritants or two problems, removing one is not going to bring you 50% of the way back to health. This is highly applicable in the world of food sensitivities. I have been recommending diets to change health for over 20 years, and it has done my heart good to see some of the recommendations that 20 years ago caused me great ridicule in the medical community to now be recommended by the most conservative healthcare organizations.

I was astounded when I saw a research article discussing eosinophilic esophagitis, a condition that is increasing in frequency across the United States, and how effective removing milk, egg, soy, wheat, peanuts/tree nuts and fish/shellfish was in treating this particular condition. I have been successfully recommending a similar diet for years for that condition, and it is good to see the academic world catch up to the clinical practice of Functional Medicine.

It really seems dangerous to me that we would prescribe a patient a high dose steroid or acid-blocking agent before we would exhaust all potential safer options. Certainly dietary changes are completely benign in the short term, and if effective, are something that can be easily and safely continued while the body has a chance to heal.

A very accessible book on this subject was written by my friends, Dallas and Melissa Hartwig. *It Starts With Food* guides the reader through the fundamentals of how food interacts with the body to create states of health or disease. This is a wonderful place for anybody to start as they go down their healing journey and question if their body and health could be impaired because of a dysfunctional relationship with a particular food.

Step 5: Retrain Dysfunctional Patterns

The next step to create health is to retrain dysfunctional patterns the body has developed.

The Question to ask here is, **"Is my metabolism, neural pathways, behaviors, immune system, or bodily structure in a dysfunctional rut?"** Patterns of bodily function that were helpful at one time may become detrimental if persistent over the long term.

The human body is a remarkable system that adapts and learns how to better survive on a moment by moment and day to day basis. Sometimes, however, it gets into a dysfunctional cycle and needs to be Retrained so it may function normally again.

One such retraining applies to the immune system as we can utilize immunotherapy to reverse allergies or sometimes food sensitivities. One form of immunotherapy is commonly known as allergy shots which are received in a doctor's office. At MaxWell Clinic we prescribe the same FDA approved allergen extracts as allergy drops which are taken under the tongue at home. These drops teach the body how to again be tolerant of substances it has developed an allergy towards.

It is remarkable to watch a person that has had a lifelong allergy to dogs or cats all of a sudden develop an immune system that can then tolerate those pets in their life. I vividly remember an 80 year old retired priest in my practice. I came in the room to do a follow-up visit after he had started sublingual immunotherapy some 6 months prior. Upon entering the room, he eagerly shows me a picture of a dog and he says, "This is my dog," and I compliment him on how well groomed the dog is, and he again says, "No, this is my dog" and he starts to cry. He repeats again and again, "This is my dog. This is my dog," with the emphasis on the "My."

The look on my face must have clearly communicated that I didn't understand the significance, and so he quickly clarified. He told me through eyes streaming with tears and a face beaming with joy, "I have wanted a dog for 70 years of my life, and now I finally get to have one. Thank you so much." Phew! That brings tears to my eyes as I write this. THIS is why I went into medicine; this is the effect of retraining a system.

The neurologic system can be retrained through the process of biofeedback & **EEG neurofeedback.** Biofeedback is a process where a signal from the body (such as heart rate or body temperature) is made conscious to the person through the use of some type of technology. This awareness creates "feedback" of how the body is functioning, and this feedback enables us to learn and change. I can now drop my heart rate and blood pressure substantially and raise my skin temperature nearly 4 degrees as a result of my retraining with biofeedback.

Neurofeedback is a special type of biofeedback where the body activity that is being monitored is the person's own brainwaves.

If we have a way to "see" our brain waves then we have the ability to change our brainwaves. This is literally "changing one's mind".

All learning is based upon the feedback of knowing if you got something right or wrong, based upon a reward being received or not. This process of learning is called operant conditioning and it is the basis of neurofeedback's capacity to train the brain to be more electrically efficient. How neurofeedback helps individuals with mood, anxiety, seizures, migraines, head injury, neurodevelopmental disorders and Asperger's are covered elsewhere in this book.

The awareness of body positions that occur during yoga is a way we can retrain our structure to function and move more efficiently to decrease pain, improve flexibility, and increase strength.

The retraining of the psychological system is approached by reconstructing an individual's narrative. This is accomplished through relationship, talk therapy and counseling. Changing the meaning of various stressors and challenges in a person's life may effectively remove those experiences as stressors.

Step 6: Reboot Set-Points

A less obvious way we support the creation of health is by rebooting.

A question of curiosity here is, **"In what ways have I accepted being stuck, and how can I regain new levels of freedom with new massive actions?"**

We have all been there. Our computer is lagging or a program has locked up and there is no hope of it working out the way we want to. It has gotten locked in a set-point. So we hit the button to reboot, to let the system recover by disrupting the non-functioning pattern and hoping that when it starts up again it will work as designed.

Rebooting only works when the instructions for proper functioning are embedded in the system. Here we go back to my personal logo and object of meditation- the Tensegrity Structure. No matter how you smash or twist it, as long as you do not break it, it will snap back to it's designed architecture. The body contains much wisdom that often gets tangled up because of the distortions of time, erosion, stress, injury, aging and decay. But if the system is at once disrupted and supported it can often break out of these set points and attain surprising advances in health.

A set-point comes in many varieties. It can be a state in our metabolism, body clock, thoughts, or electrochemistry that is our usual way of doing things. It can be thought of as a vicious cycle, a virtuous cycle, or a stagnant pattern. It is the momentum and/or inertia of our functioning. For example, some toxic metals such as lead and mercury can disable the very chemistry required for their detoxification. Similarly, refined carbohydrates may feed microorganisms that disable digestive enzymes in order to enrich their own "diet" at the expense of their human host. The problem worsens the problem.

We recognize that we have a body fat set-point that is not easily changed. Some weeks we could eat more, some weeks less, but our body fat set-point stays generally in the same area until life influences such as hormonal changes, stress levels, changes in our inflammatory level, or our sleep patterns, shift that body fat set-point. The eat less, exercise more approach certainly works within a range and for a time, but without attending to the multiple causation points of body fat production and storage intelligence, it's astounding to me how often we gravitate back towards our original set-point.

Many mechanisms of creating health can be thought of as set-point disruptors. One of my favorite things to recommend is counseling and talk therapy, or writing therapy. Telling your story out loud to another human, or out loud to yourself, can break through set-points of belief that have constrained you in the past.

Other set-point disruptors are electro-biophysical therapies such as transcranial electrical stimulation that is used to stimulate certain brain centers and put energy into the system to help that system break through a brain wiring pattern that is stuck. Other biophysical treatment strategies such as cold laser, BEEMER, TENS units, transcranial magnetic stimulation, or Ondamed, are all ways that we can put energy into the system and disrupt a dysfunctional "stuck" set-point.

Exercise can be thought of as a set-point disruptor, as can certain nutritional supplements such as sulforaphane, which is a compound found in great quantities in cruciferous vegetables, especially broccoli sprouts. It can send a new message to our NRF2 gene cassette, which will cause the body to produce more antioxidant and anti-inflammatory enzymes. Phytochemicals such as resveratrol, quercetin, curcumin, dihydroquercetin, EGCG, pterostilbene and countless others are also genetic signalers which can change our set-point of genetic expression.

Fasting is a set-point disruptor. Just not eating for a period of 12 to 14 hours changes our body's genetic expression patterns. Longer fasts have utility as well as does a fasting mimicking diet. Exercise and fasting go into the larger group of influencers called epigenetic influencers, which change our genetic set-points.

Physical intervention such as massage, body work, lymphatic drainage, an inversion table, or physical therapy can certainly break through set-points of structural stagnation. There are psychological techniques such as tapping and EMDR which can be very helpful for breaking through a set-point of anxiety or stress, or post traumatic stress disorder.

In the cognitive realm, facts can be set-point disruptors. Learning new information should change our minds. Unfortunately, in our world we observe all too often that the premature cognitive commitments of the brain are resistant to new facts, because it is easier neurologically to hold an old opinion rather than to change your mind. The inability to change one's mind is often the sign of a biologically sick brain – we know this because as the frailty of age sets in, an all-too-common characteristic of stubbornness and resistance to change also sets in. When new facts cannot change somebody's mind there may be something else going on.

At MaxWell Clinic® we are pioneering and researching what I hope will be one of the greatest set-point disruptors for creating health that has ever existed.

MaxWell Therapeutic Plasma Exchange (MTPE) is a process that removes plasma (the liquid part of blood) from an old or diseased individual. That fluid volume is then replaced with albumin, immunoglobulins, or plasma from a healthy young person in combination with specific nutritional and other health supportive factors.

In mice this process has been shown to activate previously quiet, non-functioning or dysfunctioning (senescent) stem cells in multiple tissues of old mice exposed to the plasma of young mice. This results in multi-tissue regeneration of the liver, muscle, bone sking and brain. Young mice exposed to the plasma of old mice act as if poisoned. Old plasma causes young mouse stem cells to act old, to not regenerate tissue as effectively. Brain stem cells of young mice exposed to old plasma are stunted, and some die. We will cover this more in the chapter "Infusing Hope into Alzheimer's".

Via this process there is great reason to hope that we may be able in one fell swoop to Replenish Regenerative Supports, Remove Degenerative Forces, Retrain

Dysfunctional Patterns AND Reboot Dysfunctional Set-Points.

Examine – the New Reality

After deciding upon a health-improvement course and running the experiment-of-one on yourself of Replenishing, Removing, Retraining, and Rebooting, the next important step is to pause and Examine the new reality.

Just as we started the process by Imagining the Desired State and Examining the Present Reality, now we re-enter the cycle of change and Examine the New Reality that you have created.

How you do this will depend deeply upon what your goal for increased function was, and what interventions you have chosen. Ideally, you will recheck evaluations of Body, Brain, Being, and Behavior that were abnormal at the start of your journey.

As we have detailed in the rest of this book, every person's brain is subject to incredible bias, so to combat this I favor objective measures of function. Lab tests to evaluate inflammation, hormones, metabolic function, toxicity, energy production, immune function, nutrient status and microbiome balance are all very useful. Neurocognitive tests, qEEG brain maps, MRIs, tests of vascular, pulmonary, and neurologic function help to measure the presence or absence of real results.

And just because in your current life position you cannot measure everything, do not let that be an excuse for measuring nothing. Tracking your waist circumference, your Hemoglobin A1C (a measure of long-term blood glucose) or your physical endurance are remarkable examinations of data that deeply matters for health.

Start where you are.

Imagine again – the New Desired State

It is not unusual for the initial desired state to be refined at this time. This can be because we often underestimate the power of our body to heal, and with aggressive intervention and comprehensive support we often change more than we originally thought possible.

Striving for even higher, faster, stronger, smarter, more creative, more joyful, more peaceful and more beautiful becomes imaginable with change.

If the outcome of your initial changes has not been all you desire, the question that helps us find clarity is **"How massive of an action do I need to engage that I may create health given how damaged, stuck, depleted, or toxic I am?"**

Examine again – the Process

Reassessing the New Reality is really a waste of time if that data is not fed back into awareness to further refine your strategy to create health.

Refinements may be major or minor, may involve many aspects of your forward plan for health, or may be limited to small tweaks. That is up to you, your doctor, and your larger health support team.

This is the time we also sit back to reflect upon how we are experiencing the process. Much of this process has focused upon the **Max** of MaxWell, but the **Well** is just as important.

"Well" is as you recall represented by the exhale in yoga – it is the soulful surrender into the now, the deep satisfaction garnered from the present, the joy of accomplishment and the peace of rest. To live so that you will not get sick or die may cause one to miss out on living, and that would be the very definition of counterproductive.

Creating Health is a joy to experience and to behold. Do what is Wise and Works. Commit yourself to wholesome visioning of what is possible for you, fearless examination of what is your present state, Replenishment, Removal,

Retraining, and Rebooting and continual refining of your process and experience.

Refining one's relationship to a personal MaxWell is a place of great satisfaction and accomplishment and a pursuit that is well worth the investment of a lifetime.

Part 2: Growing a Better Brain

The Center of it All

The largest challenge in the quest for real results is the necessary focus on lifestyle change. It is something that I mistakenly thought depended solely on the commitment and tenacity of the patient.

I found many of my patients were held back by their inability to make lifestyle shifts that we would agree upon during an office visit. No amount of cajoling or scolding from me was helping, so I sought out mentors in health coaching, 20 years before it had become a recognized field.

I was fortunate to find the best in the field, Drs. Mark Percival and Greg Kelley, who taught me how to approach healthcare from a principle-centered coaching perspective – one that places the choices of the individual at the center and focuses on providing the essential ingredients for lifestyle change: inspiration, education, and support.

Health coaching gave our clinic a definite edge, and I saw many patients benefit – and yet, our failure rate was still too high for my satisfaction. What was going on? I had a strong grounding in conventional allopathic medicine, which allowed me to diagnose and treat disease. I'd experienced the paradigm shift of Functional Medicine that allowed me to better understand, assess, and act upon the connectedness of function and dysfunction from a systems-based viewpoint. And we were now employing the skills of coaching people to make the lifestyle changes that are fundamental to creating health and well-being.

Why did I still see many people fail to get well when they had adequate education, inspiration, support, and resources? Why did some people do so well, while others were not able to follow the program or, despite working with counselors and coaches, could not shift limiting beliefs?

The answer came to me in part via my own pain. As I was starting up my practice, for many reasons (multiple overnight ER shifts to pay the bills of a new practice was a big contributor), I slowly and insidiously began to gain weight and become fatigued and cloudy-headed. Irritability was the norm, and headaches and ringing in my ears were an almost daily event. As my health declined, so did my brain function. As my brain function declined, my ability to pay attention wavered and my lifestyle choices began to deteriorate. One night when I had my typical dull aching headache, as I was holding my head in my hands yet again. I remember asking myself the question, **"what is this pain trying to teach me?"** And then it came to me – that Ah-Ha! moment when I realized that my problem was much like that of many of my failed patients.

At last I honed in on the answer. The brain was the problem *and* the solution. The patients who weren't experiencing leaps in wellness were struggling with attention, mood, memory, concentration, cognition, information processing, and brain speed that impeded their road to wellness. The problem was their BRAIN!

These individuals may have had great intentions for changing their wellbeing, but they were unable to take those intentions and turn them into actions. Essentially, their brain-body function wasn't allowing them to reach their hearts' desires. It turned out to be my biggest breakthrough yet. Over a short span of time, I became convinced that the brain is at the center of creating health, wellness, and the lives we've always dreamed of . . . and this is where every journey of health creation really needs to begin.

The first step in healing a brain is understanding how it works to enable or inhibit your desired state of being. This is the realm of ruts and furrows.

Ruts & Furrows

"There is frequently more to be learned from the unexpected questions of a child than the discourses of men."
- John Locke

The miracle of curiosity is that it is the antidote to the most dangerous condition in the human brain: unconscious ruts and furrows.

A rut is a track worn into existence by repeated use. On my farm in South Dakota, we have a remnant of wagon wheel tracks left by the migration of great numbers of people from east to west. Grandpa said it was part of the Oregon Trail, and I refuse to do more study to refute him.

I can only imagine how many hundreds or thousands of families passed over that terrain – each wagon pushing down a little deeper, making the path a little easier, more predictable. However, if one wanted to get out of such a rut – good luck. It caused stress on the wheels of the wagon, lots of extra horse or oxen power, and a rough ride through unfamiliar territory. It was much easier to slip back into that rut.

A furrow is a small valley formed by the first blade of a plow as it is pulled across a field. It is the trench that is formed by the blade cutting into the earth, lifting the soil, and throwing it to one side. It is very difficult to make the first pass across a flat field with a plow because there is no furrow. But once that first furrow is made, the job becomes much easier. I have spent hundreds and hundreds of hours of my life sitting on a tractor plowing fields. It is the most mind-numbing work you can imagine for 99% of the time. For 99% of the time, you keep one front tractor wheel in the furrow, the tractor in gear, and the plow fills that furrow and makes another one where your wheel is destined to reside on the next trip down the field. It is hard to get out of the furrow and very easy to stay in the furrow.

It is useful to think of your functional brain as a network of ruts and furrows. Neurons (brain cells) that get activated together over time start to associate together as a single unit. This phenomenon is known as Hebb's Law and it can be remembered as "neurons that fire together, wire together." As neurons fire together and wire together those networks of neurons become better at sending that particular signal with less metabolic energy consumption. As we will detail later, the brain loves efficiency. This firing and wiring is the basis of neuroplasticity – the brain's ability to learn and to change itself.

Ruts represent those things you have learned and with more repetition (more wagons) the less work it is for your brain to get the job done. For example, you have electrical patterns (ruts) that represent the neurology of riding a bike, or writing your name. Those activities have deep ruts, therefore efficient electrical connections, and thus do not tire out the brain at all. Ruts are easy to stay in.

Your beliefs are also embedded in electrical brain ruts that make life (mostly) more efficient. Ruts provide the benefit that you do not have to re-think "does gravity exist?" every time your foot takes a step forward. That matter has been settled and is a deep, efficient rut.

Other ruts may not be so pleasant as they may enable a near automatic fear response to a particular situation, hypervigilance, depression, or bad habits. Ruts make it hard to even attempt to see the world through another person's perspective. Ruts enable auto-pilot for good or bad.

Furrows represent those activities you have recently done, or thoughts you have recently experienced. When confronted with virgin sod, that first path the plow makes is very hard work, but once a single pass down the field has been completed it is very easy to put the front tire of your tractor in the furrow and go down that same path again and again. In the brain, it requires less metabolic energy to go down a path that has been recently traveled than to forge a new one. In other words, it is much more likely that your brain will go down the same path again and again unless there is reason not to. This is like being at a dinner party when a topic for which you had no particular opinion comes up. It is clear from psychological studies that whatever opinion you voice as you take sides in a discussion, it will be very hard to then change course later – even when new contradictory information is supplied. You have created a furrow and now it is easy to drop your electricity in that path and plow the same field again and again the same way in the future. This can be observed as people attend political rallies as well – whatever the viewpoint (furrow) of the crowd, that can quickly become the previously non-committed's furrow. It is easy to drop one's wheel into a neurologic furrow, and tough to plow fresh ground.

These networks of furrows and ruts enable your brain bias. Bias. All too often this word has been thrown around like a weapon – an accusation meant to demean and diminish the ideas of a person that thinks differently. And yes, in common use it is a negative term, a prejudice, a pre-conviction. But that is not how I am using it at this moment. Bias from my perspective is the slant, the rut, the furrows, the patterns that each of our individual brains are most electrically inclined to utilize.

Curiosity is the counterbalance necessary to prevent being trapped by one's brain ruts, furrows or biases. Questions grappled with an open mind, can save your life.

I go back to Tina, and all the other people that have died because of being caught in the brain rut of themselves, their family, or their doctor. Questioning the status quo, asking if there is more, if there is better, if there is safer, is our protection against the bias of the expert. A curious mind may save your life!

Oh yes, the person most at risk for the dangers of bias is the expert. Why? Because the person that has identified him or herself as an expert has now tied their ego – their sense of self – to what they have declared as truth. It is much harder to change your mind when your ego is attached to it.

Curiosity can protect the human from the expert. Curiosity can open possibilities for different avenues to create health.

Let's reflect upon the fact that the brain works upon electricity. Every time we have a thought, a sensation, or send the signals to create movement, electricity is created by metabolic energy being unleashed in the connections between neurons. This electricity has a tremendous cost. Our brain consumes 23% of our daily energy yet it only comprises 2.5% of our body's weight. This energy is not inexhaustible. When we use a particular brain circuit that has not been used before, or has not been used frequently, it uses more brain energy than well worn ruts or recent furrows.

People will say, "I have been thinking so much my head hurts." They will experience what I call "brain-pain." Not necessarily a headache, but a sense that "I want this to stop," a sense of being overwhelmed. This sense leads individuals to self-distract or withdraw to escape the brain-pain. Alternatively, that individual may try to push away the reason for the neurologic fatigue with anger or hostility. In short, people will exhibit a wide variety of behaviors to make the brain-pain stop. They will do anything to give their exhausted neural networks a break. This may include drugs, alcohol, addictions, violence, app-distraction, or anything that stops the brain-pain.

I believe inefficient networks of neurons are the root of most of the symptoms we call "mental illness."Individuals come to a particular state of mind as the result of many interlocking causes which may date all the way back to intrauterine development. These causes ultimately affect the electrical firing patterns of the brain. Inflammation, toxins, cellular energy production, neuronal migration, early life trauma, and lack of educational opportunities all contribute to the end wiring and firing pattern our brain is expressing today.

In the quest to help people who struggle with conditions of the brain that affects thought, mood, attention, behavior, relationships and achievement, we have thought it wise to give these people diagnoses that they may be taken seriously. Those labels are shortcut terms that help medical science by improving communication among doctors and researchers. For example, Major Depressive Disorder, can then be separated out from the rest of the human condition as a problem to be addressed with all the tools available.

However, those diagnoses often put individuals in a box called mental illness, which implies there is something wrong with them that is not their body. Many patients resist this label because they come to the conclusion that if it is not their body then the problem must reside in their soul, their very essence. Society all too often comes to the same conclusion.

Instead, we should call these afflictions what they are – Neurological Dysfunctions of multiple types with roots in Brain, Body, Being, and Behavior. Mysteries to be solved, humans to care for, not people to be merely labeled.

I love working with people dedicated to having the best brain possible because never in all of healthcare do you change a life so close to its core as when you enable a brain to function at a higher level of self-regulation.

Let's step back a moment and define a "question." A question is momentary chaos in the brain unleashing all of the potential around your brain's capacity. Electrically this is phase shift, a period where a call goes out to all centers of the brain looking for any information associated with the question at hand. The longer the phase shift, the more unique components can be brought together into a new answer.

Phase lock occurs when the electricity of the brain locks down and connects – for only milliseconds – various parts of the brain that most strongly signaled "Yes!" to the question at hand. This process of search and select, search and select, is how we work on an idea neurologically.

Said another way – when you hear a question all of the groups of neurons that connect to that question activate. All of the areas that contain the associations, the objects, the people, the places, the ideas become available to fire off together. In an operation called phase shift, the brain starts to link those various pieces together, and in a process called phase lock, the electrical activity comes into relationship.

Different parts of the brain come into relationship with each other and form a cohesive electrical pattern in your brain. This is an idea. This is an action. This is a new understanding in your brain and the opportunity that a question gives you is access to the deepest capacity of your own mind to solve a problem.

When there is an urgent need for an answer because of pain or fear, there is great pressure to resolve this chaos. To move from a brain in phase shift that is open to all of the associations and knowledge that your brain has to a state of phase lock where the flow of information, wisdom and insight creating chaos is locked down is the process of deciding. There must be phase lock so that there can be certainty, so that there can be an answer and so action can be taken.

In order to understand this neurology of changing your mind, let's briefly consider autism. The autistic brain is characterized by having very short periods of phase shift (fewer associations and new information can be integrated into the present) and longer periods of phase lock. The long phase lock inhibits information gathering from taking place.

This may explain in part how individuals afflicted with autism get "locked-in" to a particular idea, behavior, speech pattern, and why it may be very difficult for them to get out of such a pattern. We have treated many autistic children and adults in our clinic using the tools of systems medicine and neurofeedback to modify the electrical patterns of their brains and the results have been nothing short of remarkable. I think it largely has to do with shortening phase lock and increasing phase shift periods in the brain.

This concept of electrical switching helps us understand basic human behavior patterns as well. Desire is like phase shift – a seeking out for resolution, a questioning of the possibility of having something that is not yet mine. An answer is like phase lock – the fulfillment of desire.

Desire causes us to seek out that which is more, better, faster, lovelier, more wholesome, more exciting, more novel. When we are in a state of having all the answers we can give the appearance that we have everything figured out and life is not a problem. There is no chaos in our brain. There is no pain or desire; rather, we are fulfilled and have all the answers. This is a deeply seductive state, something that our brains yearn for electrically. However, it is not a state of learning or of neurologic flexibility.

So, **how do better questions enable us to live the life we desire?** Even that question in itself has triggered in your brain a desire for an answer and you are seeking it out right now. Your brain is so smart.

Humans have become the pinnacle species because we are better problem solvers. We figured out how to get out of the jungle. We figured out how to make fire, to form relationships, to create language, to distribute that language via the printing press or the internet, and to create cultures and complex rules, systems, machines, and technologies. All these things happened with a necessity or a desire leading to the question, "How could I ... ?" and the answer appeared.

Questions create health because, when faced with a health challenge, there are several responses.

One potential response is *denial* that there is a problem, that is by necessity not listening to the problem and not asking a question of how to get out of that problem.

Another way we can respond to a health challenge is by *distortion*, believing that the world is a certain way when reality says it is not.

The third potential response is *engagement.* By asking the questions we engage and harness our brain's power to transform. Some useful questions may be, **"What does this symptom, this problem, this scenario mean for me and is it what I desire? How can I improve? How can I break out of my rut and be a more full version of myself than I am at present?"**

Recognizing that our daily existence is our life experience interacting with the ruts and furrows of our brain brings the opportunity for hope. Hope that is enabled by recognizing you are in a rut, and more and better questions can carry you up and out of that rut to a new path.

The Curious Brain

"The boldness of asking deep questions may require unforeseen flexibility if we are to accept the answers."
-Brian Greene

Helping my patients thrive in contrast to merely existing is not only my job; it is my passion in life. It is the driving force behind my longstanding pursuit of optimized brain function.

Many times I have witnessed the light returning into a person's eyes after crushing depression, and the jaunty ease of an individual that waltzes into the exam room after conquering anxiety. I have celebrated with patients as grades improve, and promotions are attained as learning, memory, and attention are expressed at the level of that person's true capacity.

My eyes well up even as I am writing this, thinking of the return of a father to his family after recovering from much of the dysfunction of a head injury that occurred 20 years before. And I rejoice with those persons who experience their memory becoming sharp and dependable again after a period of decline. Brains are the most personal of organs, and the privilege I have in working with them is a privilege I do not take lightly.

An un-maximized, dysfunctional, or sick brain shows up in all kinds of ways, from the inability to focus on the things that are truly important, to the numb darkness of depression, to the exhaustion of anxiety or sleeplessness, to the devastation of dementia and the tragedy of becoming less relevant to oneself.

Brain function exists on a continuum, ranging from the maximally well – those who operate at peak performance in the present and foreseeable future – to the brain dead. All of us exist somewhere on this continuum, and where you stand is a description of your health state.

At this very moment, the state of your brain health is the result of the past interplay of your choices, exposures, experiences, and genetics, and how those choices, exposures, experiences, and genetics were shaped by countless generations before you.

Notice that of these many influences on your brain health, only genetics is out of your control. We have discussed together that human beings have an amazing potential to thrive, to maximize wellness. And I have asserted that we all have the power to improve our brains and therefore, improve our lives. But if it was that easy, would we smart humans not have already done this?

The problem is this – the very organ we are using to perceive reality is the organ that we are endeavoring to improve. We are literally trapped inside our own head.

This is quite a paradox that the following story may help to illustrate.

Imagine for a moment that you wake up from a deep sleep and find yourself inside an airplane. You're in the passenger cabin, alone, and all the window shades are closed. You feel the deep rumble of the engines, hear the whining of the wind around the cabin, and smell the stale, recirculated air.

But where you are, what direction you are traveling, and how fast you are going are questions you simply can't answer with the data you have collected. You may be able to use faint clues from what you feel, see, hear, or remember from a previous flying experience to conclude that you are, in fact, flying . . . but what certainty do you have that you are correct? Heck, you could be in an elaborate flight simulator at the mercy of some crazed operator in a remote location!

In order to assess your situation, you need feedback from your environment. Imagine now opening the window shade. Sunlight makes you squint, and when your eyes adjust, you see a familiar range of mountains (out of curiosity, what mountain range is that for you?) That's your first clue about where you may be, though of course it is subjective.

If you have the key to get inside the cockpit, objective measurement instruments such as GPS, altitude meter, map, airspeed sensor, and a compass would help fill in the blanks . . . though would you understand all those dials and gadgets in, say, an A300-Airbus? Unless you're a pilot, decoding all that data while you're in flight would likely be impossible.

In a situation like the imagined one you're in, the most helpful feedback would be an interactive call between you and air-traffic control on the ground, or at least a radio chat with a person in a similar situation in a nearby plane. The combined information from all of these sources – your passenger section observations (subjective information), the cockpit dials (objective hard data gleaned from within your plane,) and communications with other planes and air-traffic control (objective information from third parties and experts) – would help to provide you with a not only more certainty on your present location, but a safe and enjoyable journey to your desired destination.

What does this have to do with the brain? Right now, the problem is that you are trapped in your brain in the same way you found yourself alone in that plane. And without outside information, all you have to rely upon to understand your current brain functioning is your brain's own (electrical) paths of least resistance. When I asked you which mountain range you perceived outside your airplane window, it is likely that your answer was linked to either a familiar range (e.g., the Rocky Mountains) or one in recent memory or thought.

This connection is because of the "brain ruts and furrows" described earlier. These are electrical-chemical patterns in our brains that, via denial or distortion, can prevent us from maximizing the potential of our brains.

You inherently understand brain ruts because you see their effect in your everyday life. To review, your abilities, thoughts, actions, beliefs, talents, vices, and virtues are all, in essence, brain ruts. They are your practiced, familiar, conscious, and unconscious go-to responses to the world around you. The sum total of your brain ruts is your brain bias – who you are at this point in time. And, simply put, understanding brain ruts – especially your own brain ruts—is the key to healing your brain.

We have mentioned Dr. Hebb before, but now it is time to get to know him better. Donald Hebb, PhD, was a Canadian neuropsychologist who was ahead of his time. In 1949, when scientists examined the brain through the eye of a microscope, they saw axons and dendrites (the "wires" that extend out from a brain cell) and reasoned that one cell connected directly to another in a hard-wired manner. How else could the electricity in the brain be expected to flow? This became accepted dogma.

But before our microscopes were good enough to show the synapses (the tiny separations between every neuron in the brain), Dr. Hebb theorized that our brains were plastic. Not made of plastic – but flexible, changeable, bendable. He coined what has become known as Hebb's Law: "Neurons that fire together, wire together."

When neurons scattered around the brain release their electrical charge at about the same time – and they do this repeatedly to complete some action of thought, sensation, motion, or emotion – they begin to modify themselves so that the electrical pathway is more efficient for the next time that firing pattern is needed. In essence, this is why we get better at the actions we repeat most often.

Those pathways of electrical efficiency are what I have called brain ruts. The familiar is much easier to access than the unfamiliar. This is convenient if you want to remember the name and face of a work colleague, but it is through this same function that a person who has experienced a traumatic event will develop post-traumatic stress disorder; the person who went through the trauma suffers by reliving experiences long after the reality has faded.

Our patterns of electrical efficiency make up our cognitive bias – our expected way of seeing and experiencing the world.

Why is it important to pay homage to Dr. Hebb and his law? Because our awareness and brain function is limited by our current brain ruts. Brain ruts are simply electrical impulses, but they can steal our confidence and our chances of discovering and expressing our highest potential and all that makes our brains remarkable. It is very likely you have far more potential than what you are currently accessing.

The good news is that the technology now exists to enable each of us to assess and potentially escape our dysfunctional brain ruts and soft-wire new, more highly functional pathways (depending upon your brain ruts, you may have had a particular reaction to that last statement – one that could range from hope and expectation to cynicism and disdain. I ask you to be fascinated by this phenomenon of bias as you continue to read . . . and to also recognize that if you have ever "changed your mind," you have actually physically rewired your brain. Cool, huh?)

When I say that you are trapped inside your brain (and therefore your brain ruts), it may seem that I am stating the obvious, but I want to emphasize that it is NOT obvious to us that we are trapped inside our own heads; that the brain, as our organ of perception and understanding, is challenged to perceive and understand its own condition.

Just as you, a passenger in your brain-plane, cannot describe the paint job on the nose of the plane, or know whether the landing gear is down or how much gas is in your tank, you – as the owner of your brain – cannot see its functioning except by observing the impact your life has upon the world.

Another way to understand this is that it is almost always easier to identify brain dysfunctions – lapses in attention, mood swings, faltering memory, erratic behavior, underdeveloped social skills, poor coordination, bad hearing, and low intelligence – in those around us than in ourselves.

From the data we collect about other people's lives – such as their ability to reach and achieve their goals, to live productively and peacefully – we can deduce their brains' current functioning and health trend.

Each of us is a co-traveling brain-plane for those to whom we give feedback. Each of us can be aided by the words and feedback of others. When we are suffering because of an ingrained brain rut – whether it be through injury, toxicity, biochemical perturbation, genetic predisposition, or stress – and in need of assistance, we may, ironically, be the most unaware of our trouble. And without that feedback, without being curious and using all of the objective tools around us, we will not only be less aware of our current functioning . . . we will also be less appreciative of our potential function.

So, to best understand your brain function, you have to get outside of your head, so to speak. There are many ways to assess and understand brain function, and there are many approaches that can be helpful for improving it.

While it is vitally important to know your brain's present health state and what got it there, it is also important to know your health trend – is your brain learning, growing, creating an exciting reality day by day, or is it falling deeper into negative ruts?

The brain is always learning and using what it has understood in the past to build upon new revelations and today's improved functioning. When Einstein was asked what the most powerful force in the universe was, he reportedly said, "Compound interest." Yesterday's investment accrues interest, which is added to the principal, and so a small investment can become a massive fortune over time.

The brain works much like compound interest: our investments in learning, experience, healthy behaviors, and brain optimization are the foundation upon which our new potential may grow.

Remember my neuro-hero, Dr. Hebb: the more we do or experience any one thing, the more our brains will "soft-wire" that action or understanding into our networks of neurons. If we understand our brain ruts and the bias they create in our lives, we have the power to reshape and maximize the brain in profound ways.

As I hope you're beginning to see, your brain is the key to your quality of life. You deserve the best brain possible. You deserve to discover the fullness of who you are and to experience the dynamic, clear, expansive life of your dreams because of it. I invite you to accept the possibility that you are not just a passive airline passenger, trapped on a plane that's hurtling into the unknown. You are the pilot.

As the pilot of your brain, you only have one set of eyes with which to examine your brain. Because of its complexity, the brain is best understood when examined from many different angles simultaneously with expert eyes.

However, every expert you may encounter in person or online will have their own bias – their own brain ruts – on how the brain works and what it takes to improve brain function. That is not a bad thing, so long as you do not fall hook, line, and sinker that one view of the world is the end-all-be-all and therefore you do not consider other possibilities. It is a wise saying that if you find someone who has all the answers, the appropriate response is to RUN THE OTHER WAY!

Treatment plans at my practice, MaxWell Clinic®, take Brain-Bias into account by acknowledging primarily six major areas of a patient's brain health. I refer to these interacting biases as the "6-S Map" because I've found a way to describe the intricate web of brain health and the bias that both enables and impairs our healing by using a grouping of alliterative words that start with S. The idea, besides their catchiness, is that when we tug at one string of the web to intervene in a person's brain health, it invariably modifies all the other parts.

The main categories of potential Brain Bias are Soup, Spark, Setting, Story, Structure, and Symptoms. I actually have about 30 more "S's" but these are 6 biggies. So because I love diving into cellular health and metabolism, we will start with my core bias. Soup.

Soup:

If you visualize cutting open the brain, the stuff that oozes out is what I call soup. This soup contains neurotransmitters, cell membrane molecules, energy production molecules, toxins, hormones, and inflammation molecules to name but a very few.

The Soup is the biochemical component of the brain, and addressing someone's brain health through intervening with their soup recipe, if you will, is primarily done through diet changes, metabolic biotransformation (fancy word for detox), medications, and appropriately targeted, dosed and timed nutritional supplements.

This is the realm of the Personalized Systems Medicine specialist or the advanced Functional Medicine physician. Evaluations of biochemistry can be as simple as a basic blood test, or as complex as full genome sequencing, and tests of metabolism, energy production, hormone levels, chronic infections, allergies, toxin burden, nutrient levels, immune set-points, etc. Through our association with many niche labs from around the world at MaxWell Clinic®, we have the capability to test for thousands of different causes.

If you have ever heard somebody say, "They tested me for everything," you heard that person declaring their ignorance about what is possible in the world of laboratory medicine.

I am tempted to go on for days on this topic, as the interplay of mitochondrial health and brain function and the interplay of the gut-brain axis are so interesting! Toxins of many types work together to blunt our potential. Targeted nutritional supplementation has so much support and potential when examined through the eyes of fundamental physiology. Hormones and their changes and control mechanisms as well as inflammatory agents and signals have huge influences on the brain. But those will have to wait for the next book, blog, or podcast.

But know this. If a biochemical cause has not yet been found, or if there is more to the puzzle, it is almost always possible to look deeper, broader, or in another direction. Never give up – keep being curious, as there is almost always a biochemical fingerprint of dysfunction. And once a problem is understood the opportunity for a solution is greatly increased.

Spark:

The brain is an incredibly energy-hungry organ, consuming 22-25% of the energy you intake each day.

It needs this energy to create electricity, and this electricity is what we see lighting up the brain in beautiful, colorful EEG brain maps. It has been said that Psychiatry is the only specialty that does not examine the organ they treat. That is particularly sad when one realizes the technology is available now that enables such measurement to take place in your own doctor's office with no risk of bodily harm.

If you or someone you love has a brain issue, I encourage you to consider obtaining a QEEG brain map. It lends so much insight, and can direct what type of treatment may be best to maximize the wellness of that individual brain. With a QEEG Brain Map we can see the three dimensional electrical brain ruts that are present, and because structure and function are related in the brain, we are able to often show people in living color where their brain challenge is.

A remarkable Spark-centered treatment is neurofeedback – a process by which a patient's brain gets immediate feedback as to how to improve the efficiency of its own electrical flow (brain ruts). By a simple method, the brain learns how to self-adjust its electrical set-point in such a way as to help heal seizures and address ADHD.

Neurofeedback has been known to help heal a spectrum of life's brain ailments, including depression, anxiety, migraines, insomnia, learning disorders, Parkinson's, early-stage dementia, Asperger's, autism, and head injuries.

I have had the pleasure of organizing, directing, and teaching the first U.S. Medical School sponsored Brain Fitness certification program for EEG-neurofeedback and quantitative EEG brain mapping. In our office, we utilize many different software packages and hardware solutions to match the right neurofeedback programs to the right person. We even provide neurofeedback for patients that are at home.

I love neurofeedback. I get the biggest kick out of watching a person transform as their brain achieves higher levels of long term function. It is SO COOL!

Let's go more deeply into what neurofeedback is. As I said earlier, neurofeedback is the process of training the brain to be more electrically efficient so that it can function at a higher level.

Remember, neurons that fire together, wire together. This is the fundamental reality of learning. Anytime we do something repeatedly, we get better at doing it. We can train the brain to be more electrically efficient and higher performing by utilizing this ability of the brain to learn.

We start by placing an EEG cap on the patient's head so we can measure the brainwaves from the surface. This is painless, safe, and easy. At this time, we often give the patient a challenge such as pressing a button only when they should, and not when they should not. All of this information is recorded, checked for static, and then analyzed via computer to eventually make "Brain Maps."

These maps can be 2D with a series of head images on the page using color to signify if there is too much or too little of any particular wave present. Maps of how fast electricity is flowing through the brain under different conditions. 3D maps are then created allowing us to see where in the brain the inefficient waveform patterns are coming from.

Because structure and function are so intimately tied together in the brain, knowing where a problem is present, and what kind of problem is present gives us options for treatment, using neurostimulation, neurofeedback, drugs, supplements, dietary changes, or behavior change.

I contend that there is no such thing as a "normal" brain – each person has uniquenesses and I embrace those uniquenesses if they are helpful and functional for that person. However, we know what is average "normal" because we have the output of several databases of individuals that have not had seizures, head injury, psychiatric or neurological diagnosis, not on any medications, and with above average intelligence. The average of the brain patterns of these individuals is what we use for comparison when creating an individual patient's quantitative EEG (qEEG) brain map.

Once we have obtained a qEEG brain map and understand the electrical patterns present in the brain and how they may be inhibiting that person's highest function, we program a computer to assist that person in learning more effective brainwave patterns.

An EEG cap is placed on the person's head and the computer watches the brain waves that are being produced. When the brain waves that are being produced are of the type, pattern, and amount that are optimal, that person will receive a reward. If the brainwaves are not what are desired for optimal functioning, the reward is taken away. Most often, the reward that's given is the movie the patient is watching plays brightly and loudly.

When the brain doesn't do what we want it to, the movie gets dark and quiet. The brain wants the stimulation of the movie, so it figures out the three dimensional neuronal electric combination lock to turn on so that the movie will play more vividly, and because neurons that fire together, wire together, new brainwave efficiencies are trained.

What does this look like in the real world? More efficient brain waves have been shown to improve symptoms of depression and anxiety, to improve attention and working memory speed, to help individuals who have suffered head injuries, and to improve the brain functioning of those individuals with Autism and Asperger's Disorder.

It is also well documented that EEG Neurofeedback is effective in decreasing the number and frequency of seizures of many different types of seizure disorders, as well as in diminishing migraine frequency and severity. It has also been shown to improve the ability of individuals suffering from addiction to stay in treatment and stay abstinent for longer periods of time. Neurofeedback is safe, effective, and it has a characteristic of the therapies I most admire. The longer you use it, the less you need it.

If the longer you use a therapy the less you need it, then that therapy is creating true healing and optimizing function.

Some of our patients are seeking that extra edge in the business, sports or musical world (we are located in Nashville so that makes sense, eh?) To maximize their brain potential, we will utilize EEG Neurofeedback for peak performance training. We use the same technologies – but different databases and software packages – for individuals who are suffering from brain dysfunction that want to obtain a higher level of normalcy.

No matter your starting point, a better brain enables a better quality of life.

Setting:

Our brains are deeply influenced by our current environment. Brains need exercise, sleep, sunshine, sustenance, and a social life. Brain dysfunction can be caused by lack of these important ingredients.

Who you live with, your job, your school, your friends, your place of worship, and your family of origin have all shaped who you are. Some people will explain every brain dysfunction present in themselves or others in terms of their setting. And like any bias, if it traps you it is not helpful.

Stress is a real killer and the effective transformation of it can come via many different directions and resources.

Stress is a response of the body to a change in the world, but more often we understand stress as a feeling of tension or disease in our world. One of the most remarkable tricks that I can teach a patient is the trick of paced breathing. This is a simple technique where one slowly breathes in for five seconds and out for five seconds, and repeats while focusing on thoughts of gratitude. It is remarkable to see how the shoulders relax, the facial muscles soften, and a person's tension can be immediately improved.

I call this yoga 'light.' It is a simple exercise that is remarkably powerful and can be exercised anywhere at any time. I also strongly recommend meditation. This may be foreign to some individuals, and to a vastly larger number of individuals it has been something that has not been able to be accomplished. I was one of those people who just could not get into meditating. I loved doing yoga but sitting still and focusing on my breath in a way that I could deepen my practice and decrease my stress was never something I was able to do without technology.

I used our neurofeedback tools that we have in our clinic to successfully guide me to deeper states of relaxation, but I also needed access to these states when at home and traveling. A new tool has surfaced that is remarkably effective at helping meditation to be effective and enjoyable. It is called the Muse headband. It works with your smartphone. It is an easy to wear and comfortable headband that connects via Bluetooth to your smartphone. Your smartphone then drives the audio component of the experience.

This is neurofeedback light. The headset will watch your brainwaves and gives you the reward of a pleasant sound when you move into a state of deeper meditative practice. This is really a quite remarkable, inexpensive, and accessible way to very quickly deepen your meditation practice.

Story:

This S in the web is a mighty complex one, but one that I would be remiss without directly addressing. Every patient comes in with a story they tell themselves and the world about their wellness and their life.

This story is where we typically think brain bias exists (although it exists in all aspects of brain function) and it is the area that must first be conquered if you are to escape the limitations of your own brain.

If you believe that the body is destined to decay and there is nothing you can do about it, you will either do nothing or seek out experts that will tell you what you already believe.

If you have a story that you are not worth the investment of time, money, and/or energy that will be required to improve your brain function, you will likely not hear the experts who preach that you can improve if you apply yourself.

If you believe a story that your disease (e.g., depression) is caused by a drug deficiency (e.g., Prozac) rather than having multiple interacting underlying causes that can be reversed – you will seek out, and hear what your brain is prepared to hear from an expert that is singing your song and will prescribe that medication.

It is only by thinking new thoughts and asking better questions that we are made more free. Through collaboration with story experts (doctors, health coaches and therapists), I encourage you to find ways to re-frame what is possible for your life.

Structure:

One tool I have found remarkably helpful in understanding neurodegenerative disease is the volumetric MRI. This is a brain scan that maps the structure of the brain which is then analyzed by a computer and compared with a database. This database divides out the brain into different sections and compares that individual scan with a group of normal brain scans.

When a brain has been injured, or is markedly diseased it will atrophy – or shrink – in that area. Different injuries and disease processes will cause different patterns of brain atrophy. Knowing these patterns gives insight as to the cause of that person's brain dysfunction. Additionally, the clear view of areas of the brain that may have suffered large, mini, or micro-strokes gives strong evidence for blood vessel disease being a contributor to any brain related symptoms.

Some experts in the field of neuroradiology state that brain shrinkage with age is not _ever_ normal. But rather than being normal, it is common and is due to the effects of blood vessel disease in the brain. Any brain health program needs to include strategies to support optimal blood vessel health.

Fluid chambers exist inside the head, and if pressure builds up in these chambers it will squeeze the brain in a way that causes symptoms of unstable walking pattern, bowel or bladder incontinence, memory impairment, headaches, mood changes, and visual changes. If this is recognized early, much damage can be avoided.

Head injury is a far more common affliction than usually recognized. One of the most common major symptoms of a head injury is memory loss around the time of the event. This means that individuals that struck their head strongly enough to jiggle, stretch, and tear their neuron connections may be very likely to not recall that such an event happened. In cases where head injury is suspected as a contributor or cause, it is important for family members and close friends to be questioned with the patient for the occurence of concussion or head injury. I have witnessed neurofeedback transform the lives of many head injury patients.

Symptoms:

Most of conventional Psychiatry and much of the rest of medicine is based around the bias of symptoms.

The official definition of practicing medicine is to diagnose and treat patients. Diagnosis means "to know through and through" – but instead of that lofty goal, diagnosis has decayed into giving a name to a problem based upon the symptoms present.

For example, depression has become not just a terrible symptom that robs the joy of life, but instead it has been elevated to the status of being a disease. The problem with this is that there are many different causes for the symptoms of depression, and often the giving of a diagnosis will stop the process of investigation and instead trigger a this-for-that prescription of a drug marketed to treat that newly-named disease.

Let me be clear that I am not anti-drug, but I am pro-understanding the patient. When the bias of diagnosis is active, a group of symptoms will often lead the doctor to hastily apply a label of a disease which enables the quick ending of a patient visit via the prescription of a drug that is 'indicated' for that disease.

Earlier I introduced you to this, the Name-it, Blame-it, Tame-it bias of our current healthcare system. Name the disease by recognizing a pattern of symptoms, blame the made-up-name of the disease for causing the symptoms, and tame the symptoms with a chemical that almost always has unintended consequences. Seeking out the cause of the symptoms with the goal of creating health is a superior approach – but that is my bias. :-)

Finally, now that we have looked at 6 ways of looking at the brain; Soup, Spark, Story, Setting, Structure, and

Symptoms, we can easily see that none of these approaches has a corner on the truth of reality. Each person's brain problem is a mixture of these issues, and it is our opportunity to conquer the bias that traps us in our own head and look beyond our current list of available options and find a higher MaxWell.

You are now empowered to look at your brain as the organ that it is. You now know that in part your choices have been limited by the knowledge and experience your brain has had up until this point. It is time to break free.

I invite you to dig deeper and ponder the following Questions...

Is your brain performing at your Absolute Maximum Potential? If not, what kind of brain dysfunction are you currently experiencing?
(Here are some words to help you explore this idea: Joy, Motivation, Depression, Anxiety, Learning Disability, Fatigue, Insomnia, Pain, Incoordination, Memory, Attention)

_____

_____

_____

_____

_____

_____

What is your current bias when you want to describe what is wrong with your brain or the brain of another person? Story, Soup, Spark, Setting, Structure, Symptoms? Something else?

_____

_____

_____

_____

_____

_____

What one step can you take today to investigate an area of function in your brain that is somewhere unique from what you have explored before?

_____

_____

_____

_____

_____

_____

How can you start being part of your own solution?

_____

_____

_____

_____

_____

_____

There are few things more interesting than learning about your own brain, and I am honored to be on that journey with you.

Part 3: Using Questions to take on Dementia, Data and Cancer:

Rebraining Dementia

"Men ought to know that from nothing else but the brain come joys, delights, laughter and sports, and sorrows, griefs, despondency, and lamentations." -Hippocrates

Next in this book we want the rubber to hit the road. How do these different ways of thinking about health change improve real-world outcomes?

Let's start out with a very bold question. **How can we reverse dementia?**

Alzheimer's is a very scary label. To have the loss of self, the loss of memory, the loss of independence, and the loss of the ability to care for one's self is terrifying. I have cared for many patients afflicted with dementia, and I am happy to say that on a case-by-case basis, even before we had Therapeutic Plasma Exchange technology, we have witnessed the slowing of progression, cessation of progression, and reversal of dementia with aggressive intervention.

In a TEDx talk I delivered where I discussed our Systems Medicine and Plasma Exchange process to address dementia, I also reviewed some terrifying statistics: Dementia is the #1 cause of death currently in the U.K.; 18 billion unpaid caregiver hours are expended in the U.S.

every year for the care of those afflicted with dementia; nearly 250 drugs have been developed and studied for the treatment of Alzheimer's since 2003, and all of them have failed; 4 Billion dollars in research since the last approved drug.

Yet, I say there is hope. How on earth can I assert that we have hope? In order to overcome our bias that reversing dementia is impossible, we need to ask ourselves: **Is Alzheimer's any different than any other condition that we have discussed?** Is the health of the brain different in some way than the health of any other part of the body?

I would submit that <u>it is not different</u> and that, by utilizing the six steps of creating health, (Imagine, Examine, Replenish, Remove, Retrain, Reboot) we can indeed positively affect brain health and potentially cause the reversal of the degenerative process.

Alzheimer's is not a simple or a single disease. Instead, it is an end-stage degenerative brain condition named after a dead doctor. I think the term Alzheimer's should be abolished. It harms people. I have witnessed many people throw in the proverbial towel upon hearing that diagnosis and start the process of dying that day. The term itself is toxic. If it must be used it should be a verb – Alzheimering. In this way we are reminded every time the word is used that it is a process, and a process can be intervened upon.

Dementia is a better term. Dementia literally means UN-brained. There are many causes of brain loss. There are hundreds of separate toxic, metabolic, hormonal, injury, inflammatory, lack of repair, and lack of growth causes. If we find the underlying causes to the development of accelerated brain loss and address those causes, we should be able to change the trajectory of the illness. Indeed, I have witnessed it to be so many times in my practice.

As a property of my early years I have used the example of a "brain in a hay barn" for many years. It has been fun to hear this analogy being used more all the time to explain multifactorial causation.

Every farm in South Dakota had a big barn with a hayloft in the second story of the barn. It was a treasure-trove of feed for the animals in the winter and an amazing playground for a farm boy sick of the house. I played in the haylofts of the barns on both my farm and my grandfather's farm as a child. I remember taking my little pump-action BB gun up into the hayloft to shoot pigeons. I was frustrated that it was difficult to kill a pigeon with a BB gun so I brought my .22 rifle with me the next time. It was much more effective ... at punching holes in the roof of the hay barn. Oops!

I can still remember the punishment I got for that activity. It took me nearly three weeks to paint the outside of that barn, and for those entire three weeks I got to ponder just how important it was to have an intact roof to protect the valuable hay. Hay that is healthy and dry will be good for ongoing use for years and years. But all it takes is a small amount of moisture and the hay will start to rot, and the rotting process can extend as long as there is enough moisture to supply the process.

The more holes you have in the roof of the hay barn, the more water is exposed to the hay, and the more often it rains, the more the hay gets wet and the sooner the hay spoils. The brain is very much like hay. There are many different potential insults that can harm the brain, each of which can be represented by a hole in the roof. It doesn't matter if you have plugged one or two holes if you have 20. You are still not going to stop the decay. You have to plug up as many holes as you can find to be maximally effective.

We are continuing to build out an expert decision-making platform to aid physicians in finding all actionable "holes" that may be contributing to brain loss. The system acquires information from the patient's medical history, a list of laboratories investigating toxic, metabolic, and hormonal functions, an in-depth analysis of genetics, medications, neurocognitive testing, and even quantitative MRI and quantitative EEG measurements that aid in accurate diagnosis.

To date we have catalogued over 1200 individual potential contributors to the Alzheimering process. Causes and contributors evaluated may be genetic, endotoxic, glycotoxic, metalotoxic, xenotoxic, vasculopathic, sclerotic, structural, hypoxic, traumatic, nutritional, infectious, dysbiotic, aggregatory, inflammatory, excitotoxic, auto-immune, immunosenescent, energetic, oxidative, mitochondrial, atrophic, stimulopenic, catabolic, or other in nature.

Below you will see an early version of our categorization of these causes. The interesting thing is that these causes do not occur in isolation. There are complex patterns that emerge. Only after measuring multiple factors in each individual do we begin to see that person's unique constellation of causation.

The failure of our approach to date we feel is our love affair with reductionism, with a single pill for a single ill mentality. Instead we must do multi-factorial analysis of the problem and create a multi-factorial plan to address that complex problem that is Dementia / Alzheimering.

Example of a Personalized Causation Constellation for Dementing

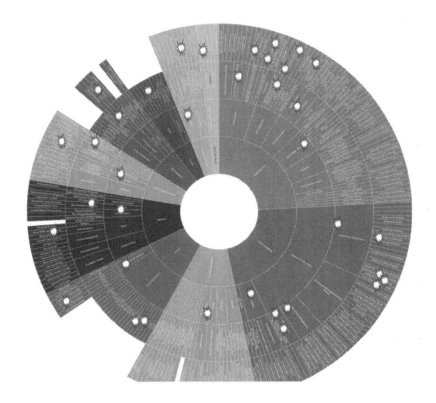

This constellation of causation will eventually be plugged into an AI engine that helps prioritize and implement this complex care pathway – creating a multi-factorial plan for the individual.

The most important people to be treated are those whom are at highest risk. The best time to plug the holes in a roof are before it has rained. It is imperative to start early and prevent aggressively – especially in family members of those already diagnosed with the condition.

This practice of Personalized Systems Medicine is the foundation for a very exciting new therapy to combat Alzheimering. It utilizes Therapeutic Plasma Exchange to shift the trajectory of illness. After reading and understanding the earlier chapters, you will see why it makes so much sense and has good reason to provide new hope!

Plasma Exchange for Alzheimer's

Of all of the chapters, this is the one I am most excited to share with you, and it took the entire book to lead up to it.

Let me tell you about a landmark new therapy we are studying to reverse the process of Alzheimering, or Un-Braining.

But first let me review what we know to be the case at present:
- Dementias (and Alzheimer's Disease as the most common form) are progressive neurologic degenerative conditions.
- The process causing this degeneration has not been understood in a way that has enabled effective treatments for these conditions to be developed. We need to approach the problem differently if we are going to hope for different results.
- We call this process Dementing, Un-braining or Alzheimering to keep ourselves focused on how this end stage condition may develop, rather than on the end stage itself.
- Un-braining/Dementing/Alzheimering is closely tied with aging. The incidence of these disorders increasing dramatically with each passing decade.
- Over 400 trials and 250 drugs in the last 15 yrs have been shown to be ineffective leading to

disappointment and despair among researchers and the afflicted. To move forward we must continue to **Imagine** a day where Dementia is conquered and Re-Braining is the norm.

- The earlier intervention is engaged in this process the more likelihood optimal brain function will be preserved. Delay in active prevention or process reversal is hastening the onset of disability, dementia and death.
- Un-braining/Dementing/Alzheimering, like aging, is currently understood to have a multifactorial causation pattern which is peculiar to each person due to each individual having a unique genome/exposeome interaction over the lifetime.
- To find the problem we must **Examine** all aspects of the systems that are contributory, from genetics to metabolomics, to lifestyle, to environment to electrophysiology to diet to microbiomics.
- These causation contributors can be understood to produce an excess of damage over repair; an excess of degenerative forces over regenerative forces; an excess of senescence over growth in the brain and nervous system. This describes accelerated aging.
- This situation causes brain tissue atrophy (shrinkage) to occur. Less brain= less brain function, less resiliency to challenge, less capacity for growth and learning, and eventual death after a long period of decay and disability.
- A systems approach to treating this dementing process would need to:

a. Identify and **Replenish** factors that are deficient that would best enable brain tissue growth, repair, differentiation, and plasticity. Such necessary resources may fall into the categories of nutrients, hormones, oxygen, exercise, light, relationships, sleep, water and purpose to name a few. Lack of resources needed to heal will thwart the body's best attempts to do so, regardless of underpinning genetics.

b. Identify and **Remove** factors that are present that are toxic, traumatic, and atrophy-inducing such as endotoxins, glycotoxins, xenotoxins, vascular insufficiency, infections, allergens and auto-antibodies. Removal of such toxic and stress-inducing factors decreases the intensity of activation of compensatory systems that steal energy and focus from the cell's mission to optimally function.

c. Identify dysfunction in genetic, metabolic and electrical patterns and **Retrain** the system to function at peak efficiency by retraining neural network inefficiencies, disadvantageous immune expression, and genetic expression patterns favoring senescence.

d. Recognize the pattern of dysfunction has inertia and intervene not incrementally, but rather as a multi-faceted **Reboot** sufficient to enable the system to find a new health-expressing set-point. Rebooting puts coordinated and robust amounts of new information, energy, signals, challenges, and resources into play simultaneously to shift genetic and behavioral expression. Effective reboots will stimulate body-wide stem cell activity and cause genetic expression patterns consistent with youth and vitality to be the new norm.

- The process of Imagining, Examining, Replenishing, Removing, Retraining, and Rebooting is the way we best enable the individual human to create health against the onslaught of degeneration
- There is one new intervention that has the potential to harness all of these routes to healing simultaneously and that is Therapeutic Plasma Exchange.
- Therapeutic Plasma Exchange has been shown to decrease the rate of progression of Moderate Alzheimers by ~60%! We believe by improving the replacement fluids used, by augmenting the process and patient care surrounding the procedure with MaxWell Systems Medicine™, we can greatly improve on this already remarkable result. At MaxWell Clinic, we are pioneering this process and investigating its application to treat and reverse Alzheimering and stimulate multi-tissue regeneration.

- We call this approach MaxWell Therapeutic Plasma Exchange™ (MTPE)

It is based upon the results of the AMBAR (Alzheimer Management By Albumin Replacement) trial which enrolled 496 patients with mild to moderate Alzheimer's disease at 41 hospitals in the U.S. and Spain and was run over 14 months. It was double-blind with neither patients nor evaluators knowing who was receiving which treatment and placebo controlled.

Individuals received an average of 18 Therapeutic Plasma Exchanges using a combination of replacement Albumin and Immunoglobulins over 14 months. Several different doses were used, but the full results of the study have not been released as of yet.

Bottom line is there was a 61% reduction in the progression of Moderate Alzheimer's disease as measured by the ADCS-ADL scale! This data was presented at the "Clinical Trials on Alzheimer's Disease" congress on October 27, 2018 in Barcelona[3].

I have also seen additional unpublished data presented and personally discussed the results with two of the Principal Investigators, Ziggy Szczepiorkowski, MD, PhD, FCAP & Oscar Lopez, MD at the annual conference for the

---

[3]https://www.prnewswire.com/news-releases/grifols-demonstrates-a-significant-reduction-61-in-the-progression-of-moderate-alzheimers-disease-using-its-ambar-treatment-protocol-300738956.html

Americain Society for Apheresis Medicine in Portland in May of 2019.

The results were described by Dr. Szczepiorkowski as "Game Changing" and indeed it is hard to see it otherwise.

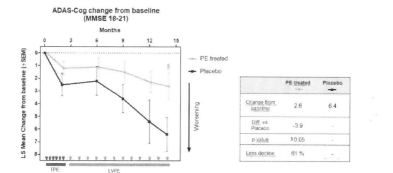

ADAS-Cog: Moderate dementia group

This study result was almost unbelievable for many individuals, but if one follows the understanding of Imagine, Examine, Replenish, Remove, Retrain, and Reboot it makes sense.

There are several outcomes with this intervention that are not ideal, but I think that is because these patients were depleted severely of nutrients and cofactors during this therapy. It was a true drug therapy – not a Systems Medicine intervention. We can do better, I believe.

At our clinic, this is how MTPE (MaxWell Therapeutic Plasma Exchange™) currently works:

We start with our Deep Dive Process, of gathering past medical information of all types, and doing extensive testing on the potential patient.

We then examine the constellation of causes that are inhibiting that person's best brain health, and create a comprehensive treatment plan. This plan includes recommendations for nutrition, activity, medications, neurotherapy, hyperbarics, IV therapy, health coaching and potentially Therapeutic Plasma Exchange, if appropriate.

Therapeutic Plasma Exchange is a well established therapy for many autoimmune and neurological conditions. It can produce a remarkable turn-around for severe life-threatening conditions where there is an excess of toxins, antibodies, inflammation, or damaging metabolic byproducts present. Does that sound useful for a problem like dementing? It makes sense to me, but it is not without risk.

Therapeutic Plasma Exchange is part of a larger field called "Apheresis" which is where blood is taken out of the body, processed, and something is returned. Apheresis Medicine is as complex as it is powerful.

Therapeutic Plasma Exchange requires an array of specialized equipment and training. In examining the utility of this approach, and understanding how it could best be applied safely I went back to my alma mater the Mayo Clinic in Rochester, MN as well as the University of Virginia and the University of California at San Diego for training and am now a qualified Apheresis Center Medical Director.

How does Therapeutic Plasma Exchange work? Two specialized IV lines are placed in the patient, and blood is pulled out of one line which leads into a plasma exchange machine. Inside the machine, the blood is mixed with a small amount of anticoagulant to prevent clotting and spun using a centrifuge to separate the liquid part of the blood (the plasma) from the red cells and platelets. The patient's plasma is then removed, and the red cells and platelets are mixed with personalized replacement fluid to take the place of the plasma that was removed.

There are many types of replacement fluids that can be used – each have known risks and potential benefits. We use our robust individualized patient data to determine what components, in what combination, with what timing are used for each individual patient.

One of the most powerful replacement fluids capable of creating health, I believe, will be proven to be the plasma obtained from young healthy donors, called young Fresh Frozen Plasma (yFFP). The collection of yFFP has many intricacies that must be followed to most optimally decrease the risk for immune reactions or the transmission of infectious disease. There is only one facility to my knowledge that holds to standards of excellence in this regard. Indeed just a month before this writing, the FDA had taken appropriate and welcome action to stop facilities and plasma producers that were, in my opinion, exposing individuals to both excessive and unknown levels of risk by their practices.

Why may it be optimal to include the plasma from young healthy donors as a replacement fluid as we are endeavoring to reverse Alzhiemering? It is because of what we have learned from the remarkable studies of Parabiosis in mice.

Parabiosis shows us a way to create health, to potentially create youth, and to reverse disease that is quite remarkable.

This is how it works – two cloned mice are carefully attached to each other by a small flap of skin on their sides. One of these mice is old, and the other young.

After a short period of time of sharing a micro-circulation, a remarkable thing occurs – the old mouse starts to show progenitor (stem) cell activation and regeneration in liver, pancreatic beta cells, spinal cord, hair, blood vessels, heart, skeletal muscles, bone (possibly), blood cells, and brain[4,5]!

---

[4] Conese, The Fountain of Youth: A tale of parabiosis, stem cells, and rejuvenation https://doi.org/10.1515/med-2017-0053

Possibly even more remarkable is that the young mouse is 'poisoned' by the old plasma coming from the old mouse. The young mouse's neural progenitor (stem) cells are stunted, and regeneration and repair is impaired.

Now do you understand why I took the time to discuss the big picture of how health is created?

MTPE for Alzheimers has the potential to create health for the brain in a way never before imagined. Never before has such a potentially comprehensive yet safe approach to brain healing been possible.

In one well-thought-out process MTPE for Alzheimers may operationalize the process of Imagine, Examine, Replenish, Remove, Retrain, and Reboot for the body so that stem cells may be activated, damaged tissue repaired, and regeneration be accomplished.

The process of MTPE is hypothesized on an individualized basis to replenish comprehensively the nutrients, growth factors, DNA signaling agents, microbiome community, metabolic resources and stimulation needed for regeneration. It will remove heavy metals, organophosphates, VOC, mycotoxins, auto-antibodies, the signals of aging, and cellular debris that are associated

---

[5] Liu, Young plasma reverses age-dependent alterations in hepatic function through the restoration of autophagy, DOI: 10.1111/acel.12708

with the acceleration of degeneration. The process will endeavor to retrain old progenitor cells to act young again and the immune system to cease it's attack on self. And finally I hypothesize that MTPE by the very nature of its massive simultaneous intervention will enable a reboot, to create an escape from multi-organ feed-forward degeneration and the potential for an ongoing feed-forward positive cycle of healthy systems interacting with healthy systems.

It is an exciting time to be a physician researcher. It is an increasingly hopeful time to be a patient or the loved one of a patient that is Alzheimering. For updates on the process go to drhaase.com/MTPE.

Therapeutic Plasma Exchange using optimized plasma from young healthy donors, I predict, will change how we understand disease and reverse Alzheimering in the process.

What kind of Doctor are You?

"Every clarification breeds new questions." -Arthur Bloch

As you may have surmised, I have been in the realm of "What's Next" Medicine for my entire career. I have witnessed the emergence of and participated in many organizations that have moved the ball forward in human health.

I became one of the first of Holistic Medicine Certified physicians back in 2000. I was a very early MD to be involved in what is now the much larger field of Functional Medicine, and was in the first class of IFM Certified Practitioners. Just two years ago, I was part of the first group of doctors to become recognized as Board Certified in Integrative Medicine. I was practicing Regenerative Medicine before it was being called that, and I was in the running to start Mayo Clinic's Complementary and Alternative Medicine program in the previous century.

All of these terms and more; holistic, alternative, complementary, integrative, functional, longevity, lifestyle, and regenerative, have clear distinctives. It goes beyond the scope of this chapter to discuss all of the differences (and there are many). But suffice it to say, just as no two people are the same, no two physicians are the same – especially once they have peeked outside of the box of strictly algorithmic medicine.

As I look forward, I am thankful that Integrative Medicine now has an established board structure and qualification path that is recognized by the established specialties. However, the core competencies of Integrative Medicine often do not include advanced biochemical & physiologic analysis, clinical bioinformatics, regenerative therapies, or advanced interventional strategies.

What is evident is that a new specialty is emerging, one that is being facilitated by all of these other forward-thinking organizations and doctors. I believe that specialty is Personalized Systems Medicine.

Personalized Systems Medicine describes the medical specialty dedicated to diving deep into knowing an individual patient by examining multiple intertwined systems, and using that wisdom to devise the safest, most likely effective treatment plan possible.

As a medical specialty, it brings together the contributions of many disciplines as a singular interwoven network. These disciplines are principally composed of computational science, systems biology, precision diagnostics, clinical bioinformatics, regenerative therapeutics, interventional salutogenesis, neuromedical connectomics, bionic augmentation, interpersonal psychology, human nutrition, and lifestyle wellness. This combination is needed to deliver the best of practical, safe, and effective healthcare. It will be the specialty of the super-generalist of the future.

It systematizes and operationalizes, "Do What is Wise and Works."

There are several trends that have become evident in healthcare that make the emergence of a new specialty inevitable.

First, we have *more data* than ever regarding human health. In my practice, we use whole genome analysis, whole metabolome analysis, quantitative EEG brain mapping, full microbiome analysis, organic acid analysis, essential fatty acid analysis, neurocognitive testing, cardiovascular testing, toxic load testing, circadian rhythm hormonal analysis with hormone metabolite analysis, advanced nutritional marker analysis, functional tests of various organ systems, along with advanced imaging capabilities. We need professional collaboration to organize this data in a way it can be both secure and broadly available for benefit for all of humanity.

The second trend is the recognition that the behavior and dynamics of *systems of biologic function* are different from the behavior of any organ systems acting in isolation. The understanding that everything in the body works together and all factors must be considered in a combined strategy is the antithesis of a reductionist approach to healthcare. When placing systems first, the physician recognizes a need for understanding the role of unintended consequences and side effects when choosing therapies. Increasing emphasis must be placed on less toxic and less potentially damaging therapies over therapies with higher risk.

The third trend is the dramatic increase in the amount and quality of *nutritional and regenerative interventions.* From stem cells to exosome therapy to growth factors and Heterochronic Optimized Plasma Exchange, the number of restorative treatments has skyrocketed. It is no longer true that once an organ seems irreparably damaged, it is truly irreparably damaged. Regeneration is now within our reach.

The fourth trend is acknowledgement that *the brain is central.* Most of this book is an homage to the power of the brain. It is where we derive our actions, motivations, thoughts, and consciousness itself – and we are beginning to understand it bit by tiny bit. We will interface with technology at increasing levels with augmented reality, neural nets, etc., and this integration will be limited only by our brain function.

The fifth trend in healthcare is that *function is now king.* The ascendency of Functional Medicine and the success of more healthcare providers looking at healthcare in terms of function rather than disease has changed the conversation forever. The father of Functional Medicine, Dr. Jeff Bland, was one of the first individuals to recognize and teach systems-based medicine even before I am aware the term systems biology or systems medicine had been used. I strongly encourage certification by the Institute for Functional Medicine as the best first step towards engaging the more data-intensive and interventional realm of Personalized Systems Medicine.

The final trend is that in the face of more and more influence of technology in our lives, *the desire of humans to be deeply known as individuals by another human* is growing. This trend is not only the anchor for Personalized Systems Medicine, but it holds the secret ingredient of the best healthcare possible.

What is the secret ingredient of the best healthcare possible? I believe it is a very old fashioned ingredient. It is something not given as much press or encouragement as the new fancy test or the remarkable technology. It is the old school *doctor/patient relationship*.

This is a sacred relationship in my mind. I took an oath upon completing medical school to be a physician to the very best of my ability. To care for my patients in a way that I would always place their best interest first. I cannot tell you the satisfaction and joy that I experience as I, together with my patients, work to solve the human puzzle of MaxWell, right alongside of the technological, biological and electrophysiological puzzles.

With an increased interest in examining meaning and purpose in life, more physicians are seeking to re-engage patients who are dedicated to maximizing their wellness at a higher level in a personal, professional, proactive, and participatory way. Personalized Systems Medicine seeks to deliver the tools necessary to bring deep data into real patient care to better treat multiple interacting causes of dysfunction in the context of a renewed doctor-patient relationship.

Maslow's hierarchy requires our basic physiological needs as well as our need for safety to be met before we may proceed toward fulfilling our psychological and self-actualization needs. If there is not safety in a relationship, then it's very difficult to go to the next level of development and human thriving.

The doctor/patient relationship is the single best place to give a platform of deep opportunity for the ultra high achiever, deep safety for the chronically oppressed and depressed, deep hope for the person that has failed to launch, and deep investigation and intervention for the seriously ill complex medical case.

No matter what medical needs or desires a person has, they are first of all a person deserving of the highest level of dignity and respect and dare I say it, love. That, I am certain, is part of being The Good Doctor.

MaxWell Systems Medicine™ is our unique expression of Personalized Systems Medicine at MaxWell Clinic®. It is our particular vision of the new medical specialty of systems medicine that undoubtedly will be constantly evolving to better enable *The Good Doctor* to meet the needs of the patient for the creation of health and the treatment of disease. It is the best descriptor of the medicine I want to see exist for everyone.

MaxWell Systems Medicine™ is a dynamic structure (much like a tensegrity structure!) which has several tenets – the interconnections of which make a whole field. This specialty is defined not by what organ system, practice philosophy, or treatment options it includes or excludes, but rather by its dedication to determining and implementing the most direct, safe, and effective route to maximum wellness for any given individual.

It is a trademarked term so that we can deliver assurance that those physicians that call themselves MaxWell Systems Medicine™ specialists will have acquired the training, tools and experience to deliver a consistent type and level of service.

Deep Dive at MaxWell

"The boldness of asking deep questions may require unforeseen flexibility if we are to accept the answers."
-Brian Greene

Our clinic has many providers. Each has the core knowledge of Functional Medicine and MaxWell Systems Medicine™ but also has their own unique strengths and interests. We serve a broad variety of problems and individuals, from auto-immunity, to chronic fatigue, to addiction, to depression, to neurodegeneration – and the list goes on. A systems based approach to creating health is applicable to many disease states and health problems.

But what if your desire is to **live at the maximum potential of your capacity**? **What if your goal is, like one of my patients, "to live forever?"**

As part of my personal practice I have a Deep Dive investigational medicine program where we explore the limits of and develop the tools for our take on Personalized Systems Medicine. This practice-in-a practice is comprised of a small group of individuals who have committed to invest the resources of as much time, as much money, as much focus, and as much energy as is necessary to achieve their goals of performing at their highest capacity and living as long as they can at their highest capacity.

Each Deep Dive program is customized to the individual. We focus on that individual's goals regarding their particular health challenges or threats. These individuals may come to us with prior diagnoses for which they want more options for treatment. They may alternatively desire an in-depth proactive search for their health risks and a clear plan of action to change their future health story.

With our current technology, we have an immense opportunity for health and life promotion. The goals I expect from this group of people are reasonable, but also extraordinary. This program is not for somebody that is passive, or whiny, or expects health to come to them outside of any effort on their own. This program is for people who are proactive, determined, and who shape their world according to their desires.

We keep the number of participants very small because I have committed to thinking about every single person on this list every day. Whether I am out lecturing physicians on how we can create health, or sitting at my computer doing research, or out on a walk in a contemplative state, every person in this program has a daily share in the real estate that is my brain.

What may be included in an Investigative Medicine Deep Dive? We start with a very thorough understanding of who you are as a person through an in-depth personal interview. We then seek to acquire and review of all of the old medical records of your life that we can get our hands on. This includes an examination of previous laboratory studies, radiologic studies, pathology reports, and specialist referrals. After this information is acquired we have our first personal visit which is partnered with a detailed physical examination (something that often gets neglected in more rushed practices).

We couple all of this with biologic investigations looking at whole metabolomics (which is measuring greater than 700 molecules in your blood at one time), whole genomics (depending upon the situation and appropriateness of that evaluation), whole connectomics (which includes a map of your brain's electrical activity), and potential imaging studies to survey the health of your organs and structural system.

We utilize over 25 research laboratories from around the world and seek to find the data necessary to put together the patient's story in a cohesive, functional way. It is investigative medicine and it brings me great joy to get to do this.

Putting together huge amounts of historical data about a patient does not assure the best decisions possible are made. It is also very important to track the response to all interventions to see if we are making progress in the only realm that matters – the realm of real-world results.

Additionally, according to the complexity of the case and the depth of the desires for health and longevity, we will engage research specialists from around the world, medical subspecialists, and create a virtual private medical center around the patient as an individual.

The individuals who choose to do this depth of analysis to promote their own health and well-being are dedicated world changers, and it is an honor to assist them in their quest to be the fullest versions of themselves.

Our Deep Dive clients range from individuals who dedicate all they have in the world towards recovery from a serious illness, to the rich and famous that see the work we do as advancing science for the interests of society at large. Indeed with every patient that enters this program our data aggregation, analysis and extrapolation of that data improves. Every Deep Dive client also enables several micro-grants for patients in need to access the unique diagnostic and therapeutic resources of MaxWell Clinic®.

The MaxWell Clinic® Deep Dive is our endeavor to raise the bar to the best of our ability as we continue to develop and deliver MaxWell Systems Medicine™.

We also have partner clinics (and will be adding additional qualified collaborators) that are dedicated to this same ideal of using deep data to drive better healthcare outcomes. The more highly-curated and contextualized health data we can accumulate the more we can figure out "what works for whom and when." These insights will in turn improve health outcomes and decrease overall healthcare costs.

This work, to enable people to experience the full realization of their health potential, is my life's calling. Yet, there are only so many hours in the day and no one doctor can serve everybody. Thus, I have dedicated myself to making the maximum impact I can with a smaller number of these deep-dive patients and teaching doctors and overseeing other clinicians at the MaxWell Clinic® so they may move forward in the art and science of creating health.

Questioning Cancer

"If you live the questions, life will move you into the answers." -Deepak Chopra

How do we cure cancer?

This question must be answered. Cancer destroys lives, hopes, dreams, and opportunities. It rips apart families as it eats a person alive from the inside, out. It is a great evil on every level. It is hard to detect, hard to know what treatment is best, and hard to monitor if that treatment is effective.

In a quest to find better answers, we were the first clinic in the United States to offer a new test from Germany that I believe will revolutionize the detection and treatment of cancer. This simple blood test may enable the cure of cancer, much like the blood test for the HIV virus transformed the treatment of AIDS.

What changed the world of HIV? It was the development of a blood test that could measure viral load. Before, the viral load test, treatments to change the course of the disease were evaluated by waiting and watching the patients to see if they improved or progressed on to the multiple horrific stages of AIDS. With the existence of a viral load test, the iterative process of drug development and testing was able to accelerate tremendously. Lives were saved, misery was diminished. Yay, Science!

This is how the new test from Germany works: Every time a cell dies, its DNA will be broken down so the raw materials can be recycled. Some fragments of the DNA are released into the bloodstream where they can be collected. Cancer cell DNA is often filled with mutations in which big portions of the DNA molecule have been duplicated or deleted. We call these copy number variations or when measured in total "copy number instability" or CNI. The greater the amount of cancer DNA in the bloodstream, the more Copy Number Instability (CNI) will be present. This is the CNI score. The higher the CNI score the more tumor DNA is present and being released into the bloodstream. The CNI is a measurement of our Tumor Load much like the HIV test was able to measure Viral Load.

We are all developing cancer on a daily basis. Our cells are constantly being assaulted by toxins, ultraviolet radiation, and insults of one type or another. Our immune system does an amazing job of identifying these rogue characters and eliminates them with incredible efficiency, however, on occasion a cell slips through our defenses and begins to replicate, growing and mutating as it grows.

I think the CNI test is an excellent candidate to be a single-blood test cancer screening tool, however more data is necessary before we can depend upon this test alone. The remarkable thing about this cancer test is that we, for the first time, may be able to understand how much cancer we have in our body at any one time. Our tumor load.

The CNI may therefore be one of the best cancer tracking tests available. There is not yet enough data to use it as a sole marker for cancer load surveillance, and it is still an investigational-use-only test. However, its accuracy in matching the clinical course of many patients I have tracked over the last 3 years has been uncanny.

One of the biggest problems with cancer therapy at the present time is that it's very difficult to run trials to know what works for a particular patient in a timeframe that is optimally helpful for the individual. Once a cancer is diagnosed, it requires complicated scans and biopsies to understand the characteristics and pervasiveness of the tumor. Once this understanding is reached, the patient is assigned to a treatment algorithm based upon very limited data compared to the amount of data that may be potentially acquired. Treatment is then started and we wait, and wait, and wait until either the person dies from the chemotherapy, tolerates the treatment well only to find that the tumor has progressed on the scans, or tolerates the therapy to make it to their follow-up scans and biopsies to get the verdict if the last three, or six months of hell was effective in decreasing the tumor burden, hopefully, to the point of eradication.

A recent study published in Clinical Cancer Journal revealed that by using before/after sampling, this CNI cancer test was able to provide an 83% overall prediction accuracy in predicting response to immunotherapy and disease control/progression, with a positive predictive value for progression of 92% after one cycle of immunotherapy. After a second cycle of immunotherapy, the CNI-score yielded a 100% positive predictive value for progression. Six cases of hyper-progression were observed, five of which could be identified by the CNI-score at a significantly earlier time point than by the current practice of imaging (six - nine weeks earlier). One patient with progressive disease who had been misclassified as stable on the basis of imaging assessments was able to be diagnosed correctly by the CNI score[6].

Other data shows that testing before and after chemotherapy was able to predict if that therapy was going to be successful at three or six months of therapy after only one or two courses of therapy had been administered. This means we can know if the cancer is responding to the therapy long before the previous toxic waiting time between three or six month scans.

MaxWell Clinic® is a pioneer in this domain by virtue of my connection to the research world. I was asked to give

---

[6] Tumor Cell-Free DNA Copy Number Instability Predicts Therapeutic Response to Immunotherapy, Weiss et al . CCR 2017. The publication can be searched on http://clincancerres.aacrjournals.org/content/early/recent

feedback and advice to the company that developed the CNI tumor load test as I care for individuals that are highly committed to maximizing their wellness. It has been astounding to watch the CNI numbers drop as successful therapy has been administered. And it has been heartbreaking to see ineffective therapy for patients create an increasing number of unsuccessful results. The numbers go up as a therapy is proving ineffective for a person. It is remarkable to see the vast genetic uniqueness of cancer cells and how this uniqueness can be used to track how much cancer is present in the body and how much of its DNA is being released into the bloodstream.

Obtaining the test is rather simple. The blood is drawn and we extract the free-floating 'scrap' DNA from the plasma. That scrap DNA is then replicated and the Copy Number Instability (CNI) is measured. The more damaged DNA is present indicated by a high CNI score, the more likely there is a tumor present. And because we can map the types of DNA mutations represented in the CNI, we will gain a better understanding of how to target therapy forward going.

All that being said, I still do not believe this test should at this time completely take the place of any existing tumor screening, but it may serve as an adjunctive screening test in the context of prevention. Additionally, the potential risk of emotional distress, economic burden, and possibly excess medical diagnostic procedures is a real risk when using this test if the result is high and after a tumor search has been completed nothing has been found. Informed consent is critical before engaging in any diagnostic or therapeutic endeavor, and all the more so in the realm of advanced surveillance.

This tumor-load test is one example of many different advanced testing capabilities available in the world (at least at MaxWell Clinic). Other advanced testing examples are whole genomics (your genetic blueprint), metabolomics (the interplay between your genetics and environment), whole transcriptomics (what your DNA is doing), immunomics (what your immune system is reacting against, etc.). These advanced testing capabilities are available in part because of our Deep-Dive program and all patients at MaxWell Clinic have access to them.

You can find out more about this methodology at www.DrHaase.com/cancertest.

Part 4: Questioning Supplements

Nutritional Supplements?

"It is error only, and not truth, that shrinks from inquiry."
-Thomas Paine

Why is it that nutritional supplements cannot treat or cure disease? Answer: Because the FDA says it is so.

Interesting fact: The very definition of a nutritional supplement includes in that definition that it cannot treat or cure or prevent disease. If it could treat or cure or prevent disease that would *by definition* make it a drug under the FDA's definition.

So, nutritional supplements are required to claim that they do not treat or cure or prevent disease to stay out of the categorization of being a drug. It doesn't matter how many studies, how much science, reason, or personal results are experienced, the nutritional supplement may never claim to treat or cure or prevent a disease based upon this technicality.

In some ways this is just silly and it is a way of not speaking honestly on many levels. I have witnessed nutritional supplements be instrumental in the process of creating health for individuals. Oftentimes, these individuals get so much better that they 'lose' their diagnosis (but let's not call that a cure - ha!).

On the other hand, the technicality is brilliant because disease is more of a human made-up-definition and therefore is not something that is as addressable as a definable metabolic dysfunction. Understanding what the biologic dysfunctions are that cause the body as a whole to not work is way more important than putting a fancy name on a really bad illness. Understanding always outdoes opinion, even if the opinion is that of an expert.

I used to be radically anti-nutritional supplement. I thought that we could get everything we need for optimized health through food. And then I realized nutritional supplements were concentrated food. I began to understand how ridiculous I was being by having a prejudice against a food that was put into a capsule form in order to increase its availability, its palatability, its stability, and the effective concentration one could ingest in a reasonable amount of time.

Nutritional supplements as concentrated foods are incredibly safe as a class of substances, the major side effects coming almost entirely from the group of fringe products that extreme weightlifters consume to jack themselves up or products that are contaminated with drugs, toxins, or illegal hormones.

"If you're not up on it you're down on it" is a statement all too true in the realm of nutritional supplements and modern healthcare. Because the amount of information to know is dizzying and the internet information sources are questionable at best, a good and cautious physician will often defer to the position that if he or she cannot know what is in that product, or what the science is that justifies its use, then he or she should not recommend it, and I would say that is good medicine.

Every trained physician has probably watched somebody die or knows that in some way they have participated in the demise of a patient. Caring for sick people is tough business in the best of conditions and circumstances. To help ease suffering and cure disease, physicians have occasionally advocated things that in the end have turned out to be very harmful. Drugs such as Vioxx, DES, Thalidomide, Trovan, or Rezulin all have a place on the wall of shame, and many doctors prescribed these compounds to the detriment of their patients.

This is absolutely NOT why physicians go through medical school, and work ridiculous hours under demanding circumstances. My physician friends are some of the best humans I know – very caring and compassionate people that never want to be part of an error. These experiences appropriately encourage physicians to be highly conservative when it comes to doing new things. The fear of the unknown around nutritional supplements often causes physicians to not engage in that route of therapy with their patients. I have found that this is only out of lack of information.

Having spoken with thousands of physicians from across the US and around the world, I am struck that the vast majority of them take nutritional supplements, and when they feel assured of the quality of the source of the materials, they prescribe them for their patients.

I am currently the Medical Director for XYMOGEN, Inc., one of the largest professional supplement companies in the United States. Having had nearly 20 years experience in this field and having helped formulate many products, I can say with great certainty that there are a tremendous number of products that can not be described as anything other than trash in the marketplace. There are also some remarkable compounds, formulations, and supportive tools to help proactive patients enable health. All of the good, the bad, and the ugly are present with nutritional supplements. Quality control, supply chain management, and transparency are key if you are going to voluntarily and repeatedly bring a substance into your body.

I think it's absolutely laughable as I remember back in medical school when one of our pathologists was deriding the idea that taking a vitamin could be helpful. He stated the only thing that a vitamin could do would be to give you expensive urine. The idiocy of this statement still blows my mind. Did he believe that the food he ate had no purpose? Hardly. It is obvious what food does on its way through the body is exceedingly important and absolutely some of those products are going to come out in the urine. Additionally by that same logic, one should only need to take a drug to treat high blood pressure one single time because it should do its job to fix the problem with one pill. Anything more than a single pill and you're having expensive urine from a pharmaceutical.

Vitamins and minerals, plant substances, essential fatty acids, and compounds that stimulate the growth of healthy bacterial populations, as well as probiotics, all have necessary functions in the body. The ability of our body to be filled to optimal levels with the raw materials essential for life is an incredible opportunity we have in the modern era through nutritional supplementation.

Unfortunately, the use of nutritional supplements has largely been thought of as an insurance policy rather than a precise therapeutic tool. After engaging in whole genome analysis and whole metabolome analysis in my practice, I can tell you that the biological individuality of persons is incredible and the idea that one size fits all from a nutritional medicine strategy is completely out of date.

Targeting the right formulas at the right doses in the right timing for the right reasons for any individual is an art that is rapidly becoming a science via advanced metabolomic testing and computer analysis. But no matter how precise the recommendations, if the label does not match what is in the bottle the potential for benefit is lost due to poor quality or deceptive practices.

What about Supplement Quality?

"No one is dumb who is curious. The people who don't ask questions, remain clueless throughout their lives."
-Neil deGrasse Tyson

How do I know my nutritional supplement is high quality? This is a big question and it's a very important question to ask if you're going to bring a substance into your body on a regular basis. A small amount of toxicity in a product that you are taking on a regular basis will build up to substantial proportions over the course of time. Likewise, a product that is counterfeit, contaminated, low quality, or of the wrong composition can be detrimental as well.

When the supplement on the label isn't in the bottle or a toxin is present in the bottle that is not declared – THAT is where the idea of expensive urine really does apply.

What kind of questions should you be asking as you evaluate nutritional supplements?
1. Certification of where it was manufactured – process & production capabilities
2. Independent quality checks on raw material suppliers – purity & potency
3. Ingredient composition, dosing, encapsulation, packaging – quality & clinical utility
4. Storage, Supply Chain management

Since there is far less regulation of nutritional supplements than pharmaceuticals, the buyer must beware. At the top of the list in understanding supplement quality and safety is understanding WHERE the product was produced. The factory itself will tell you a lot about the quality control of the process, the ingredients, the storage, and the people behind the products being manufactured.

Certifications are often used for marketing purposes. If certifications mean anything, they should be designated by a qualified official organization that actually visits the factory being certified. There are lots of pretty slogans and decals and "certifications" on supplement bottles but many of them are easily obtained by paying a fee, or heck – you can even create your own!

In my opinion, one of the top certifications that means something is TGA Certification from the Australian government Department of Health: Therapeutic Goods Administration (TGA). If the facility from where you are getting your nutritional supplements is certified by TGA, you can know that your supplements are being manufactured at a top-tier facility.

The TGA regulates pharmaceuticals and nutritional supplements alike. It is considered to be one of the toughest regulatory agencies in the world and its inspection certification is conducted at the pharmaceutical standard. This certification is accepted by many other governmental agencies across the world. In Australia, supplements are regulated by the TGA as "complementary medicines." There is not a distinction between supplements and drugs. In order to pass certification, a manufacturing facility has to demonstrate the highest quality control procedures, laboratory procedures, and standard operating procedures.

Another reputable certifying organization is the National Sanitation Foundation (NSF). While not as rigorous as TGA, NSF inspects facilities to ensure that they do not store substances which are banned from use by competitive athletes. If a banned substance is not allowed in the building, it is unlikely to appear in a product 'accidentally.'

Organic Certification for manufacturers from the USDA assures that there are processes in place to keep organic foods under strict quality control. This assures the supplement buyer that organic means organic and there was not a bait-and-switch in the production line to increase profit margin at the expense of the consumer.

International Fish Oil Standard (IFOS) is a meaningful independent standard for measuring the potency and purity of fish oil. One thing I like about this organization is that they test the final product once it has been placed in a bottle. It is a much more realistic quality test than testing the raw material as many things can go wrong during manufacturing.

There are other organizations that will offer to certify manufacturers and products, but a fair number of these other certification bodies are not far from worthless. They will be more than happy to put a seal on your particular supplement because you have paid them a fee to fill out a checklist, or maybe have just paid them a fee.

What information should we know about raw materials? Raw materials that go into nutritional supplements vary widely in their quality and composition because, at their heart, nutritional supplements are supposed to be concentrated foods. They are meant to be digested, they are natural so they decay. There is not the ease of standardization and measurement that is present when one is evaluating a drug made of a single molecule that is not subject to decay.

Quality control in the world of nutritional supplements is very difficult because a raw material needs to be qualified in many unique ways. The specifications of precisely where the raw material originated, how it was collected, how it was processed, how it was stored, who handled it, how it was packaged in bulk, and how it was transported to the facility should be readily available. Raw materials should be quarantined in the factory until they are certified as potent and free of allergens and contaminants.

A good example is curcumin, a very popular extract of turmeric. A publication in the journal Integrative

Medicine revealed that a substantial amount of the curcumin available for sale in the United States was extracted using a carcinogenic solvent[7]. There is no place on the label where this is required to be disclosed. Many people take a supplement of curcumin thinking they're doing good things for their brain, decreasing inflammation, and decreasing their risk of cancer. Instead, they are sucking down residual carcinogenic solvents on a daily basis. This does not need to be the case. There are raw material forms of curcumin extracts that are highly validated, pure, and the entire supply chain is transparent.

I recommend curcumin products that use the raw material BCM-95 because the quality control on all aspects is tightly regulated by the manufacturer. However, it's much cheaper to buy a compound that has not had the additional cost of testing, more precise extraction processes, and a lower quality raw material. In the world of nutritional supplements unfortunately you do not always get what you pay for, but if you don't pay you may justifiably be suspicious you are not getting the best.

Supplements may be contaminated with pesticides and herbicides, so understanding where that supplement came from with regard to it being organic is important. Yet, some compounds may not need to be organic because they have never been exposed to pesticides or herbicides in the

---

[7] Liva, R. "Toxic Solvent Found in Curcumin Extract," *Integrative Medicine*, 9:5 Oct/Nov 2010

first place. In these cases, organic is often used as a marketing term rather than as a meaningful term.

It is also important to know if the raw material was derived from genetically modified organisms (GMOs) because some individuals have a higher level of allergenicity from plants that have been derived from GMOs. Additionally, GMOs are often exposed to higher levels of pesticides.

The extraction process of the active compounds of herbs and foods will give very different compositions in the end product. Understanding the composition of an end product is what standardization is all about. One of the marks of a high quality supplement is a disclosure of the standardization of that extract on the label. A common herb used to support adrenal health and neurologic function is rhodiola. A high quality product of rhodiola can be standardized to approximately 3% rosavins and 1% salidroside. However, there are products on the marketplace that claim up to a 15% to 30% concentration of rosavins. That is not a natural product in any way shape or form. What you are consuming is a product that has been spiked with synthetic active ingredients. This may be no different than taking a drug and is certainly not in the spirit of using nutritional supplements wisely.

Raw materials, once they are received need to be qualified. Qualification means the compounds are tested for potency using techniques of High Performance Liquid Chromatography, Mass Spectroscopy and DNA analysis.

During the qualification process, testing for purity also takes place. Testing makes certain there are no appreciable amounts of lead, cadmium, arsenic, mercury, or residual solvents present. Testing is also done to assess the presence of yeast, mold, E. coli, staphylococcus, salmonella, and overall potency.

Materials are quarantined during this time of testing and are only released into the warehouse for use once they have been through all appropriate testing. The raw materials need to be stored in temperature controlled warehouses or refrigerated storage for more sensitive materials such as probiotics.

It is preferential to use raw material suppliers that have had a long track record of supplying potent and pure raw materials on a regular basis. Once a supplier has delivered a batch of raw materials that is determined by independent testing to not be of the stated potency or composition, or to contain toxins, pesticides, herbicides, or other noxious compounds, not only will that batch be returned but very likely the relationship with that particular vendor should end. There are few places where the term "buyer beware" is more true than in the world of nutritional supplements because there are so many potential pitfalls present during the selection, manufacturing, processing, and distribution process.

The facility should be temperature and humidity controlled 24/7 because humidity and heat are the best way to cause natural products to rot. The miracle of refrigeration changed food storage forever in the modern world. If probiotics or sensitive compounds like SAMe are being processed, the facility should be brought down to an even lower humidity such as 15-20% as XYMOGEN is capable of doing.

As large tubs of raw materials go through machines that put the powder into a capsule, all appropriate safeguards to prevent contamination should be utilized. This may include using closed systems with gravity feed.

The powder itself must be composed in such a way that it blends to uniform consistency and flows evenly so that the correct amount goes into each capsule. This is why it's important to use safe and nutritionally beneficial flow agents to enable capsules to be consistently high quality. Some of these compounds include MCT oil, magnesium stearate, dicalcium phosphate, silica, microcrystalline or cellulose. These ingredients are found in most every meal that is eaten and come from components in the natural world.

As a sideline, it is down right silly how some manufacturers will use the presence of magnesium stearate as a negative marketing tool. Stearate is a fat that is present in vegetables, meats, and is ubiquitous in the diet. It stimulates healthy mitochondrial function.

To show how misguided it is to complain about magnesium stearate as a potential negative ingredient in supplements, consider an article from the July 2015 publication of the journal *Nature*. In this article, it was shown that stearate is important in turning on the human transferrin receptor 1 gene and supporting normal mitochondrial function. Stearate is a vital mitochondrial regulator. It inhibits the human transferrin receptor 1 activation of JNK signaling[8]. This then enables the mitochondria to function to make cellular energy more efficiently. Stearate is clearly shown to be an important molecule which regulates mitochondrial function in response to the diet.

If you'd like more information about this, I have an article posted on my website at DrHaase.com/magstearate. You can download that article, and see how this whole ingredient drama came to be. This kind of storytelling is what makes the nutritional supplement industry look incompetent and therefore, creates friction that is not beneficial to addressing more important matters.

Another question to ask about supplements is: Was the finished product tested? It should be tested for its ability

---

[8] **Nature,** 2015 Sep 3;525(7567):124-8. doi: 10.1038/nature14601. Epub 2015 Jul 27.

to disintegrate and dissolve. The specific weight of individual capsules should be identified. During processing, every bottle should be checked for metal fragments using an electromagnet detector. Finished products should be tested to make sure that they meet the label claim to at least 100%. They should be tested again for microorganisms: Yeast, mold, staphylococcus, E. Coli, and salmonella. And then checked again for heavy metals: Lead, cadmium, arsenic, and mercury. When you work with a physician to obtain your supplements through XYMOGEN, you will have access to the certificate of analysis for all recommended products.

Stability testing is not required for dietary supplements and I think that is ridiculous. If a supplement company puts an expiration date on the bottle, they are supposed to have stability data on that actual product. This is either stability testing in real time with a bottle being put on a shelf and being tested again after one to two years or whatever the expiration date is, or using an accelerated stability chamber where the increased heat and humidity are present to simulate the passage of time in a more rapid way. Many companies do not do this stability testing.

There are very clear guidelines for doing this testing to ascertain the stability of a product. Be cautious of products that have a "manufactured on" date, or a "born on" date, or a "packaged" date instead of an expiration date. Those terms are used because there is either no data yet available for stability or, more likely, stability testing is not being done on that particular formulation. By using one of these designations, the company only needs to certify that label claim was met by the product on the date of manufacture, not for any foreseeable time in the future even though that is when the product will be consumed.

Do you know where your supplements have been stored? With XYMOGEN all products are shipped straight to the patient or to the doctor's office. There is no time other than the brief period of shipping where bottles are not climate controlled.

If you purchase online from Amazon or other retailers, you may not know where that product has been stored and you are unlikely to find out its entire supply chain. Some of Amazon's warehouses have been documented to get up to 120 degrees – that is not an acceptable storage condition for a natural product. Heat will cause degradation. Buyer beware.

What is the best way to decide what nutritional supplements are right for you? This is one of the most common questions I am asked by my patients interested in maximizing their wellness. I am proud to be able to help my patients focus on the compounds and products that may be the most beneficial to them given their life circumstances, their genetic predispositions, their medications, their nutritional absorptive challenges, and their desires for performance. This is absolutely not a place for one-size fits all medicine. Rather, it is a place for the very best of customization and personalization.

The best place to get high quality recommendations for nutritional supplements is from a highly qualified practitioner that knows both you and the world of nutritional supplementation. I would also recommend you purchase your supplements from that practitioner if they make them available because details of product composition, brand, and delivery systems do matter.

For example, the dose and composition of different forms of magnesium serves as an example here. Magnesium oxide, magnesium citrate, magnesium glycinate, magnesium bisglycinate, magnesium threonate, magnesium malate, magnesium taurate, are all different forms of magnesium, each with particular strengths and weaknesses.

Magnesium oxide is very challenging to metabolize and it is a very tiny molecule. Magnesium oxide is used in cosmetics and in the making of cement. It is one magnesium attached to one oxygen, which accounts for its small size. If you want to make your label look like it has an impressive amount of magnesium, you use magnesium oxide. However it is very unlikely that this form of magnesium will be absorbed by the body with anywhere near the effectiveness of magnesium that is attached to an amino acid which is called a magnesium chelate. And even the type of chelate matters with raw materials being fully reacted (as is the case from Albion minerals) and those that are just mixtures of magnesium and amino acids without the needed bonding. A particularly useful and unique chelate is magnesium threonate which has data to support that it penetrates through the blood brain barrier and stimulates new neuron growth better than other forms of magnesium.

There are many details and a well trained clinician that knows both you and nutritional supplements is the best way that you can assure you are getting the most from your healthcare dollars for the promotion of your well-being.

To find a practitioner that is authorized to distribute XYMOGEN supplements, go to www.xymogen.com under "Patients" and "Find a Practitioner."

If you are a practitioner that wants to provide the highest quality products in the industry, go to www.xymogen.com under "Practitioners" and "Register with XYMOGEN." Not all who apply are accepted as you must have qualifying licensure.

Part 5: Making Curiosity Work for You

Who is the Right Doctor for Me?

With all of the complexities of healthcare it is difficult for patients to know the qualifications of the medical provider they are entrusting their health to.

For now, <u>there are several questions I think each patient should ask of anybody they are going to engage in their health journey.</u> There are many right answers, and you as the patient get to decide what those right answers are.

1. Do you have a license to **practice medicine?**
2. If not, what are you legally **licensed** to do?
3. What are your **certifications** of training?
4. What is the **authority** of the certifying organization that gave that certification?
5. What is your **life experience?**

Why is a license important? Because licensure is a fundamental standard of legally-binding oversight for professional behavior. It provides accountability, and hopefully protects the public from rouge egos and ignorant brains.

A license to practice medicine allows an MD or DO to legally diagnose and treat a patient. Bequeathing a diagnosis (this is what is wrong with you) and prescribing a treatment (you should do this) is the legal domain of the practice of medicine. I do distinguish this from being a "doctor" as that term is used broadly now, and in some ways has lost its meaning. When somebody says they are a "doctor" – the appropriate next question is, "What are you a doctor of?" Again, I am a strong advocate for clinical diversity – medical doctors have caused a lot of suffering in the world and do not have the corner on truth. Many voices are needed as we seek to improve the health of our world and MANY of those are not medical doctors. The patient can only benefit by knowing the individual scope of practice, strengths and differences of the members of their care team.

The Institute for Functional Medicine allows several types of licensed medical professionals to go through its certification program. The prior training those individuals have is important to understand as that license (DC, PA, APRN, RD, etc.) will deeply shape how those practitioners practice. If they do not have a license to practice medicine, they are going to apply that learning to practice functional wellness or functional health.

Next, look into what the certifications your potential provider has and what do they mean. After you have figured that out, you need to decide if they match your desires for your care. A trend is to note one's IFM certification, a dash, and one's degree associated with licensure. For instance, my certification for being a practitioner certified by the Institute for Functional

Medicine is IFMC-MD, a registered dietician would be IFMC-RD, a doctor of chiropractic would be IFMC-DC, and so on.

Also, certifications are only as good as the organizations that oversee those qualifications and training. If the organization was created to espouse the ideas of one central leader, or if the most important qualification is that you have a check that will clear the bank – then those certifications may be held in suspect.

Life experience is something that is near impossible to quantify, but is tremendously important as you choose a care provider. Their story informs the kind of diagnostic breadth, investigational depth, presuppositions, and passion that will be part of your health journey together. Ask questions of a personal nature. I love being a real human with my patients, and it is my failures and life experience that guide me as much as my knowledge as I seek to deliver care.

There are many more questions you will want to ask as you choose your healthcare team. This was not meant to be an exhaustive list at all, but a list of questions that I think too few people are aware are important.

In all of healthcare, it is unfortunately *caveat emptor* – buyer beware. We each need to ask good questions to make it more possible to obtain the help we need.

Is it Functional Medicine or Functional Marketing?

Over the last 20 years, I have practiced and studied alongside a brilliant, caring, and visionary group of clinicians and scientists assembled at the Institute for Functional Medicine. This organization birthed the term "Functional Medicine" over 30 years ago to describe a heuristic of applied systems-biology medicine and root-cause-analysis in clinical care. It is a beautiful way to practice.

I am proud to be one of the early physician IFM members, to have been certified with the first cohort of IFM-Certified Practitioners, to serve as a member of their core teaching faculty both domestically and in the international education arena, and to be the external Faculty Lead for the Energy Advanced Practice Module of their certification program.

I think the Institute for Functional Medicine sets a high standard for professionalism. They have created a great certification course to teach the foundations of systems-based thinking in healthcare. I highly recommend this certification to medical professionals looking to grow personally and professionally.

In the early years, each Functional Medicine practitioner came to this field with different histories, practice experiences, licensure, interests, opinions, and styles. There are vast differences in training, approach, practice experience, and credentials within the concept of Functional Wellness and Functional Medicine.

Unfortunately, IFM did not choose to trademark or defend the trademark of the term "Functional Medicine" which they germinated. This did not matter for my first 12 years with them because there were few practitioners and little public awareness. Then, with increased awareness of the unique effectiveness of this approach in clinical medicine, there arose copycat organizations and teaching programs all selling "Functional Medicine" – often with materials directly plagiarized from IFM. If these programs produced accurate, high quality control content, or if they were judicious about who was allowed to use the term Functional Medicine, then there would not be a problem today confusing practitioners and patients alike.

However, at present there has been an unfortunate dilution in the meaning of the term Functional Medicine. The IFM approach to Functional Medicine is a specific approach taken to patient care and applied through medical education. Some individuals want to catch the wave of opportunity, sometimes for product marketing purposes over medical excellence. Others feel that Functional Medicine simply means recommending supplements instead of drugs or doing nutrition testing.

That is so very far from the truth of true Functional Medicine.

Some "programs" that are labeled as Functional Medicine or marketed by people claiming to be practicing Functional Medicine are little more than product promotion opportunities, designed to garner a social media following or drive a sale.

Why I am spending time discussing this? Because we often see patients in our practice that have spent a lot of money, time, and effort, without getting impactful results, following generic directions and taking advice from non-medically-licensed "experts" before they make their way to our clinic door. All too often, these individuals feel jilted and angry about their experience now that they know better. They don't understand why some individuals call themselves Functional Medicine practitioners/providers, when they are not medically trained, or are not staying within the scope of their licensure.

What makes me even more sad and concerned is imagining all those individuals that have been down that path of holistic, functional, integrative healthcare, and had a bad enough experience to never re-engage their health in that way again.

Let me be clear, I have no worries about these non-licensed or questionably trained individuals being "competition," as there are more than enough people struggling with their health in the world. We are facing a pandemic of chronic disease stemming from poor lifestyle and environmental concerns. Vast numbers of health advocates can all stay busy for lifetimes educating and managing patients, the real question is how do we handle this responsibly as a healthcare community putting the patient's best interests in the center.

I have coined this click-bait friendly, hyper-promotional, opportunistic, reductionistic bastardization of Functional Medicine as "Functional Marketing." It makes me sad to witness any mailman, cyber-marketer or unlicensed course graduate of a dubious program claim to "practice Functional Medicine." This dilutes to absurdity a noble movement.

Medicine is a term that in most states is legislated to be limited to the engagement of a professional with a license to practice medicine. I think the state licensure boards should take seriously the misuse of the term "Medicine" for marketing purposes by non-licensed individuals. I see no reason for restriction for terms like "Functional Wellness" or "Functional Health," but to use the term "Medicine" if one is not licensed to practice medicine is deceptive and out of one's scope.

True Functional Medicine does not sell a pill for an ill, or manipulatively promote that "everything starts in the _____" or "your _____ is making you fat and tired" or "your genes make you _____" or "the secret is to only eat _____ and don't eat _____ and your _____ will be cured" or "the fix for your low/high _____(insert gland here) _____ problem is _____."

Unfortunately, marketing is best when it is reductionist and boiled down to a sound bite. Rarely can a sound bite accurately describe the complexity of a wholesome approach to healing the human system. If it sounds too good and simple to be true, it might be "Functional Marketing."

What is *Functional Medicine* as defined by the organization that coined the term and developed the original concept over 30 years ago?

> The Functional Medicine model is an individualized, patient-centered, science-based approach that empowers patients and practitioners to work together to address the underlying causes of disease and promote optimal wellness. It requires a detailed understanding of each patient's genetic, biochemical, and lifestyle factors and leverages that data to direct personalized treatment plans that lead to improved patient outcomes.
>
> By addressing the root cause, rather than symptoms, practitioners become oriented to identifying the complexity of disease. They may find one condition has many different causes and,

likewise, one cause may result in many different conditions. As a result, Functional Medicine treatment targets the specific manifestations of disease in each individual.

https://www.ifm.org/functional-medicine/

When I am asked where one can go to find a doctor that practices with a similar philosophy as me, I will encourage a visit to the website for the Institute for Functional Medicine, www.ifm.org, and search in your area. Examine all the licensure, credentials and experience of the individuals to make an informed choice that suits your needs and view of the world. If possible, choose a practitioner that is an IFM-Certified Practitioner (IFMCP) as it shows a level of dedication and depth that simple membership in the IFM does not.

Thanks for letting me vent a bit. I desperately want the whole of medical practice to shift to a more wholesome, systems based approach, and posers create harmful distractions that thwart the progress that could be made.

MaxWell Questions List

Below are a group of questions I have enjoyed asking over the years. They are magical questions as they will enable you to better create health.

It has been an absolute joy to write this, for you my dear reader. I hope you have more wisdom and context to now go forth and be a better advocate for your own health. I am confident in your brain's ability to serve your well-being, so long as you keep it flexible and active with good questions.

Wishing you a life of being MaxWell,

David Haase, MD

www.drhaase.com
www.maxwellclinic.com
www.creatinghealth.com

Now here are your questions of power....

If I were the highest version of myself, what would that look like?

_____

_____

_____

How would I feel?

_____

_____

_____

What would I be doing with my life?

_____

_____

_____

What's holding me back from being the highest version of myself?

_____

_____

_____

What am I doing about that?

_____

_____

_____

What kind of new resources do I need to bring into my life?

_____

_____

_____

What kind of stressors, traumas and toxins do I need to remove?

_____

_____

_____

Who do I need to live for?

_____

_____

_____

What dream am I pursuing?

_____

_____

_____

Do I feel stuck? If so, why?

_____

_____

_____

Am I living my life for something else that doesn't care about me?

_____

_____

_____

Is my current state of body-brain-being leading to the level of impact that I desire to have?

_____

_____

_____

What is my greatest health fear?

_____

_____

_____

What am I doing to address that?

_____

_____

_____

What currently held beliefs are holding me back?

_____

_____

_____

What statements have people told me about myself that have no basis in objective truth but rather exist only in their self-serving subjective perceptions?

_____

_____

_____

How am I taking over my life?

_____

_____

_____

How am I refusing to be a victim?

_____

How much power does that give me?

_____

How is my brain helping or hindering me?

_____

What is Wrong with me?

_____

How do I Enjoy Life?

_____

How can I Be Productive and be at Peace?

_____

What role does relationship have in health?

_____

How do we reverse Alzheimering?

_____

_____

_____

How may we better detect and treat cancer?

_____

_____

_____

How can we live forever?

_____

_____

_____

How do we eliminate heart disease?

_____

_____

_____

How can I maximize my brain's potential?

_____

_____

_____

What is the Good Doctor?

_____

_____

_____

What Creates Health?

_____

_____

_____

What Maximizes Wellness?

_____

_____

_____

About the Author

David Haase, MD is a doctor, teacher, and innovator who is deeply committed to maximizing wellness one unique person at a time. Dr. Haase received his medical training at Vanderbilt University and completed his residency in family medicine at the Mayo Clinic in Rochester, Minnesota. He is board certified in Family Medicine and Integrative Holistic Medicine and is among the first practitioners to be Certified by the Institute for Functional Medicine. He is the founder of MaxWell Systems Medicine™.

Early in his clinical practice, Dr. Haase knew that something very important was imbalanced. He realized his training had been dominated by an almost exclusively pharmaceutical approach to managing disease and focused little on how to instead create health. To fill the void he sought out additional medical training and certifications in nutrition, integrative and holistic medicine, functional medicine, health coaching, neurofeedback, systems biology, genomics, bioinformatics, precision medicine, and apheresis medicine.

By identifying and treating the unique root causes of their conditions, Dr. Haase feels deeply privileged to have witnessed remarkable improvements in his patients' health. Dr. Haase treats a wide range of conditions and has special expertise in brain-related disorders such as dementia, fatigue, mood, anxiety, insomnia, Parkinson's, seizures, head injury, inflammation and immune dysregulation. His friendly manner, enthusiasm, and humor make learning fun and light the way for a patient's healing journey.

Dr. Haase is the founder and Medical Director of MaxWell Clinic®, which was established in 2003 with offices in Clarksville and Nashville, Tennessee.

Dr. Haase is co-founder of The Food Initiative, a non-profit organization that helps youths make healthier choices for their bodies and their communities (www.thefoodinitiative.org). He is the Medical Director and Chair of the Medical Advisory Board for XYMOGEN, a leading professional nutraceutical company. Dr. Haase serves on the board of Evoke Neuroscience, a company providing clinical technologies to optimize brain function, has served as a consultant for Metabolon the world leader of metabolomic evaluations for precision medicine, and Illumina, innovator of Whole Genome Sequencing technologies.

Dr. Haase is a sought-after lecturer and teaches internationally about the root causes of disease and innovative, safe treatments through his faculty position at the Institute for Functional Medicine and as past adjunct professor at the University of South Florida, University of Miami, and Western States University.

Dr. Haase integrates nutrition, metabolomics, neuroelectrophysiology, genomics, environmental factors, and lifestyle medicine to help his patients get better and he shares these concepts with other medical professionals for improved patient care. Dr. Haase is passionate about making better health accessible to all people and uses his innovation and creativity to bring new diagnostics and treatments to the medical field for the betterment of medicine and health.

Please visit www.drhaase.com to catch Dr. Haase's latest podcast, blog, or just plain fun musings.
Visit www.maxwellclinic.com for information on becoming a patient of Dr. Haase or one of the other remarkable physicians or practitioners.
Visit www.thefoodinitiative.org to discover and support a very worthwhile organization.

Be MaxWell.

Curiosity Heals the Human

46213342R00135

Made in the USA
Middletown, DE
25 May 2019